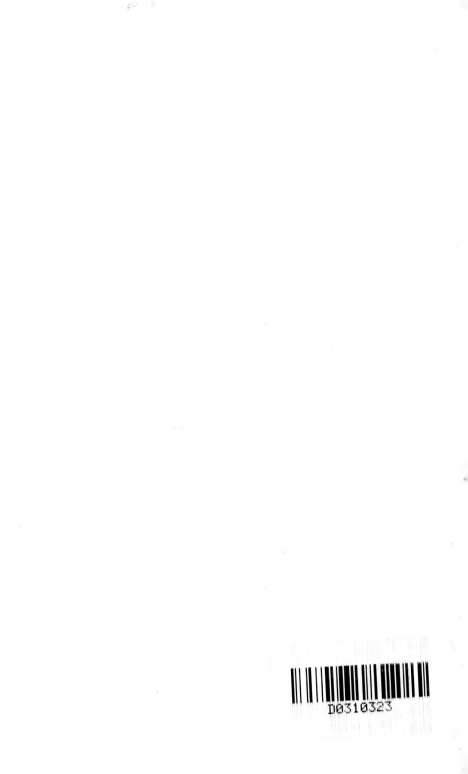

BELLA FIGURA

ALSO BY KAMIN MOHAMMADI

The Cypress Tree

BELLA FIGURA

How to Live, Love and Eat the Italian Way

Kamin Mohammadi

BLOOMSBURY PUBLISHING
LONDON · OXFORD · NEW YORK · NEW DELHI · SYDNEY

BLOOMSBURY PUBLISHING
Bloomsbury Publishing Plc
50 Bedford Square, London, WC1B 3DP, UK

BLOOMSBURY, BLOOMSBURY PUBLISHING and the Diana logo are trademarks
of Bloomsbury Publishing Plc

First published in Great Britain 2018

A catalogue record for this book is available from the British Library

ISBN: HB: 978-1-4088-5620-8; TPB: 978-1-4088-9603-7; eBook: 978-1-4088-5619-2

2 4 6 8 10 9 7 5 3 1

Typeset by Newgen KnowledgeWorks Pvt. Ltd., Chennai, India
Printed and bound in Great Britain by CPI Group (UK) Ltd, Croydon CR0 4YY

To find ... ry.com

For Old Roberto
— the tortoise to my cypress —
who would have loved to see himself in print

CONTENTS

CONTENTS

Tutto quel che vedete lo devo agli spaghetti.
Everything you see, I owe to spaghetti.

Sophia Loren

PROLOGUE

She walks down the street with a swing in her step and a lift to her head. She radiates allure as if followed by a personal spotlight. She may be tall or short, slim or pneumatically curvaceous, dressed discreetly or ostentatiously — it matters not. Her gait, her composure, the very tilt of her head is an ode to grace and self-possession that makes her beautiful whatever her actual features reveal. She is Sophia Loren, Gina Lollobrigida, Claudia Cardinale, Monica Bellucci. She is the Italian woman glorified on celluloid and on the nightly *passeggiata* you see on your Italian holidays — but she is no figment of the ad-man's imagination. She is real and walking the streets of every city, town and village in Italy right now. She is the embodiment of *bella figura* and she cuts an elegant dash through our mundane modern world.

When I arrived in Florence, I could not have been further from this ideal. Decades of working at the computer had rounded my shoulders, years of looking down into a laptop or phone had slackened my jawline and compressed my neck. The stress of a demanding job and big-city life had hardened my features. My eyes were fixed to the ground as I hurried through life, with no time to throw anyone a smile let alone a kind word. Single for years, my loneliness had calcified. I didn't so much strut with confidence as cringe down the street.

A year in Florence – and discovering *bella figura* – changed my life.

The concept of *bella figura* is about making every aspect of life as beautiful as it can be, whether in Rome, London, New York or Vancouver. It is a notion at once romantic and practical. It encompasses everything we do, from what we eat to how we get to work in the mornings. It's about sensuality and sexuality. It's about banishing the stress that, no matter how few carbs we eat and how vigorously we exercise, means our bodies are so shut down we can only ever look harrowed and pinched. *Bella figura* is about generosity and abundance, not meanness or deprivation. The Italian woman who lives the *bella figura* knows the importance of beautiful manners and a graceful demeanour, not as a nod to a by-gone era, but as a means of 'making the face' until it fits – it's a proven fact that if we smile genuinely often enough, we release the happy hormone serotonin. All of this improves not only our quality of life but also the quantity of years we have.

While this book will touch on details about already well-documented benefits of the Mediterranean diet, what follows in these pages is, instead, the story of a journey. Ten years ago I moved to Florence quite by accident, and that first year I spent there changed my life, my body and the shape of my heart. I believe that what I learnt can change yours too.

I

JANUARY 2008
Festina Lente or how to slow down

Produce in season: blood oranges
Scent of the city: woodsmoke
Italian moment: my flat is in a palazzo!
Italian word of the month: *salve*

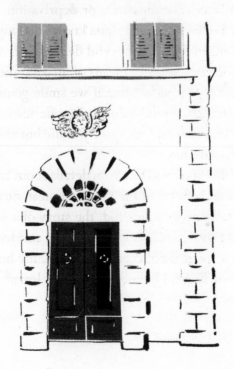

It all began with rain. It fell in heavy sheets as I was lined up waiting for a taxi at Santa Maria Novella train station in Florence. The queue was not under cover and I didn't have an umbrella. By the time I got into the cab, I was soaking wet.

I was in a city where I didn't know a soul, unanchored from work, friends and family, a piece of human flotsam washed up in its Renaissance gutters. All I had, clutched in my damp hand, was the address of the flat where I was to stay. As I reached the top of the line, I uncrumpled it, showed it to the cab driver and got in. He grunted and pulled out, frowning at the puddle forming at my feet behind him.

We swept through the slick cobbled streets. The heating was on full-blast and my sodden coat was fogging up the cab. I peered through steamed-up windows at the stone walls of ancient buildings rising up on either side of the road, water dripping off their deep eaves. The streets were deserted – it was 2 January and the city was still sleeping off its hangover. My own New Year's Eve had been spent stuffing boxes into corners in my parents' flat under the beady eye of my mother, who said nothing but whose every breath asked me what on earth I thought I was doing, giving up a good flat and a job so prestigious it came with embossed business cards to move my possessions into her already overcrowded apartment and flit off to Florence to play at being a writer. I may as well have announced I was going to Italy to run a brothel.

The cab driver slowed down, gestured to the left and grunted. I turned round to take in the majestic proportions of a colonnaded piazza, a cathedral looming up at the end of the square, its white façade reflected in the glistening ground. My mouth fell open.

It wasn't just the beauty of the square, but the theatricality of it too; the way the eye was led to the façade of the church. *'Si chiama Santa Croce,'* the driver said. Then indicating the statue of a scowling man, he said, *'E quello li è Dante.'* Dante looked as grumpy and bad-tempered as my cab driver, yet I was cheered. The man credited with inventing the modern Italian language in his *Divine Comedy* was standing right there, holding a book in his stony hands, looking at me with his basilisk stare. It was a good omen.

The basilica stood solidly behind Dante's statue, the entire square constructed to induce awe in the insignificant human approaching it, as well as delight and marvel in the beauty. It was my first brush with the perfection of Italian presentation, the importance of the harmony of form, the genius of the impact on the onlooker, the moral weight given to beauty. It was *bella figura* embodied in stone and marble.

We crossed a nondescript bridge. This time the cabbie pointed to the right where the Ponte Vecchio squatted over the river on low arches. Lit up against the night, its row of matchbox shops hanging over the water, it shimmered like a dream. I took it in, wide-eyed, as we drove on, swinging into the Oltrarno, the other side of the river Arno from the historic centre, winding through cobbled streets to pull up at my new front door.

'*Eccoci*,' the driver said as he heaved himself from his seat. I paid and stepped out straight into a puddle. I hurried into the entrance hall, taking in its cavernous proportions as I dripped on to the flagstone floor. A flight of wide stone stairs twisted off to the right and I lugged my bags up, stopping to rest on a narrow bench on what felt like the 108th floor, panting. It was still a long way from the top. The steps dipped in the middle, worn by centuries of feet: the building dated from the seventeenth century, the silence thick with ghosts. I resumed my climb and finally stood in front of a Tiffany-green door, its paint cracked and curling. The lock was a massive iron box with a large keyhole – fortified, ancient. I pulled out an equally antiquated-looking key and opened the door.

A long corridor with a rough stone floor stretched away from me. It was freezing, my breath fogged into the air. Halfway down I found a dark bedroom with two single beds and an enormous wooden chest of drawers where I dropped my bags before going back out into the corridor to find the heating, switching it on, shedding my wet coat and grabbing a blanket and wrapping it tight around me.

The flat, which would be my new home for who-knew-how-long, was stuffy as well as cold. The corridor opened into a chain of rooms linking one to the next, what interiors magazines call a shotgun apartment: a sitting room with large, shuttered casement windows, a sofa bed and a rickety table with haphazard piles of books. A long and spacious kitchen led off the top of the sitting room, the sink, cupboards and oven ranged along the right while, on the left, a table sat under another set of double windows.

At the far end of the kitchen, another sitting room was set at a right angle, with a long corner sofa behind which a shelving unit was wobbly with stacks of books. In the far corner, the only door in the whole flat apart from the front door closed off a small bathroom.

I regarded myself in the mirror above the sink: my hair was frizzy from the journey, there were shadows under my eyes and I could see the glowing red mark of a new spot erupting on my chin. Or chins, I should say. My Big Job had made me hate my reflection. The years had been marked by inexplicable, distressing, weight gain: rolls appearing not just around my middle, but on my back, under my face, hanging from my upper arms; I tried every healthy diet going and eliminated every kind of bad food as identified by the latest fad to no avail. Acne, which had given me a wide berth when I was a teenager, came to get me with gusto; my skin had broken out. I tried not to care, but the industry I worked in made that impossible – a glossy magazine company in which the daily lift ride required nerves of steel, a pre-season designer wardrobe and the insouciance of Kate Moss. I had draped myself in black shapeless clothes instead and avoided the lift.

I sighed and turned away, going back to the window in the kitchen. In spite of the cold and the rain, I threw them open and leant forward, peering into the darkness.

Outside a dark, silent courtyard was overlooked by windows, balconies and terracotta roofs. On the far side watching over it all was the tower of the local church, a slim stone structure from the seventeenth century. Four green bells peeked through small arches, a jigsaw of brickwork around the top the only decoration. All around, the windows of the other flats were dark. Rain fell into the silence.

Christobel's tower, I thought, remembering the first time I had heard about it.

I had met Christobel when I accepted a last-minute invitation to a holiday at a friend's home in France. Christobel was another guest. She had white hair with a stripe of black running down the middle, and a diamond that glittered in the corner of her nose. An unlikely look for a fairy godmother, but then, Disney never dreamed up one as sassy and smart as Christobel.

I learnt that she was a novelist, a wife to a Cambridge academic and mother to five children. She told me how she had fallen in love with Italy when she had spent a year in Florence teaching English. She had travelled back regularly, and somewhere along the line had bought a flat, talking dreamily of a courtyard and a church tower. She managed a visit most months; two days in which to be alone, no children tugging at her skirt, to wander the streets visiting her favourite haunts for cappuccinos, for designer frocks and handmade shoes. She wrote it all into thrillers set in the city, her characters retracing the steps she took around town, her plots imagining the dark underbelly of the place she loved for its beauty but was compelled by for its mystery. She had published three novels and was working on her fourth. I couldn't imagine how she fitted it all in. 'I have a full-time job and a cat, and I still can't figure out how to wash my hair during the week,' I had said, and, laughing, we had bonded.

Lying under an olive tree one hot day, Christobel had suggested that I retreat to her flat in Florence to write the book I dreamt of undertaking. I had scoffed at the time – it was a lovely dream but as far from my reality as could be. After all I had a Big Job anchoring me in London, I was far too busy to take off like that.

And then, in just a few months, I had lost my Big Job and been evicted from my flat. Even my cat had deserted me, climbing out of the window one day never to be seen again. As if she had sniffed out my despair, Christobel rang me one winter night, as I sat among my boxes. At my news, she clapped her hands in delight. 'So now there's nothing to stop you going to Florence in January to write,' she said and started making plans before I had agreed. So I had taken the hint life was emphatically giving me, drawn a deep breath, packed my book proposal and stepped off the edge of the cliff. A cliff with a Renaissance face, but a cliff nonetheless.

Now somehow, just a few months later, I was here on a one-way ticket, sitting by her tower, gazing down on to her courtyard. A ripple of panic ran through me: for the first time in my adult life I didn't have a job, an income, a flat of my own. I looked across at the tower – not just any old church tower, but where Michelangelo had once hidden from his enemies. I headed to bed.

The next morning, I was woken early by the sound of church bells. Pealing exuberantly every fifteen minutes, they foiled my attempts to turn over and go back to sleep. Light bounced off the white walls and high slanted ceilings crossed with thick beams of wood. It hurt my eyes. Large terracotta tiles the colour of wet sand covered the floor, rough on my bare feet. The heating, which had been on all night, was finally breaking through the chill.

I made a cup of tea, setting the kettle to boil on the hob in defiance of all the moka coffee machines lying dismantled on the draining board. The sky outside the kitchen window turned from pale blue to gold and then to azure as the sunlight crept down the tower, turning the cross on top aflame before bathing row after row of biscuit-coloured bricks in its glow, illuminating the grooves on their surfaces.

There was a window immediately to my left, set at a right angle to mine. It was so close I could have leant into it. This must be Giuseppe's window, the artist neighbour Christobel had spoken about with particular fondness. I could just make him out in the dark interior, stalking about his flat dressed in a thick orange fleece and a dark orange puffy gilet. With his red glasses and tawny hair, Giuseppe looked like a burst of sunset moving about in the gloom.

I positioned myself with my back to his windows to preserve both our privacy – I was in no mood to make friends just now.

I sat, letting the scene soak into my eyes until the day was so bright, the colours so rich, that I could sit still no longer. I threw on everything at hand, slipped my notebook into my handbag and clattered down the stone stairs, swung open the heavy wooden doors and stepped out on to the via di San Niccolò.

The street was narrow and overhung on both sides by tall buildings – coloured beige, cream, mustard, turmeric – the line of rooftops as squiggly as the smile of the toothless old man shuffling past. The buildings were all Renaissance like mine. Their eaves reached out over the pavement, bottle-green shutters thrown open to the sunny day, washing lines stretching between the windows. Opposite there was a bakery, windows hazy with condensation. Kneeling by the front door, a short, thickset woman with an apron was scrubbing the doorstep with a wide brush, her black hair held back with a white cap. Two old ladies walked by arm in arm. One had blonde hair teased into a meringue while her shorter friend's mass of burnished red curls were piled on top of her head. They were probably a hundred and fifty years old between them, but they were made up and well dressed, their low heels clicking on the cobblestones. They pulled shopping baskets behind them, the wheels bouncing noisily in their wake. They paused to greet the scrubbing woman, who stood up laboriously to chat, opening the door for them to step into the steamy bakery as mopeds buzzed past and people called out to each other as they headed to a café on the corner of the street. I followed them in.

The raucous sound of an Italian pop station blared out of Café Rifrullo while a flat-screen TV on the wall flick-ered with pop videos. I was hit by a wall of noise and the heat of bodies. People called out their orders, one row of bodies stepped forward as short black coffees were set down on the bar. They added sugar, stirred twice, quickly drained the coffee, then stepped aside as those behind came forward and repeated the steps. There were three baristas moving quickly behind the bar, commanded by a large black-haired, moustachioed man who dominated the bar with the same authority Pavarotti did La Scala, singing snatches of arias as he made coffees. When I finally inched my way forward, the Rifrullo Pavarotti landed in front of me. He held my eye while singing 'La donna è mobile'. Timidly, I asked for a cappuccino and pointed hopefully to a croissant. Pavarotti laughed heartily and I felt like a fool.

I took my breakfast outside as everyone in the bar stared. I cringed under their gaze but stepped out into the cold January morning anyway, compelled by the English need to soak up the sun at any given opportunity, and I settled myself, shivering slightly, on a bench to offer my face to the sun. Opposite the side door of Rifrullo there was a pizzeria, a tiny wine bar, and a swish-looking deli. Above all these, more flats in spice-coloured palazzi, two stories of windows fanned by open shutters. This short street led to a small square to the left where cars were parked at anarchic angles with mopeds squeezed in between, encircled at the far side by a crenellated wall, grass sprouting through the worn bricks: an intact part of the medieval city wall into which was cut the large open arch of the city gate of San Miniato. It was the same soothing sand colour of my tower and its crumbling surface had protected the city for centuries.

I sipped at my cappuccino, savouring its perfect mix of bitter coffee with creamy frothy milk. When I was a child, one of my favourite aunts would sometimes pick me up from school and take me to a sophisticated café in Tehran – full of intellectuals wreathed in cigarette smoke – to drink café glaces – a concoction of coffee, milk and vanilla ice cream served in a tall glass long before frappuccinos were a glint in a marketing man's eyes. I had been addicted to coffee ever since and now smiled to think that here I would never have to drink a bad coffee again.

After my coffee, I followed via San Niccolò round a corner and found the plain façade of the church, its tower – the guest star of my kitchen window – set somewhere behind, invisible from where I stood. I placed my palms on the vast iron ring handles, moulded by centuries of hands, and pushed open the heavy wooden doors as Michelangelo must have done, seeking refuge. I too had run away as surely as if I had tied up my belongings on a stick carried on my shoulder.

The cool interior was disappointingly plain, not a fresco in sight. I took a pew and thought gloomily of the career that had turned sour. And I also allowed myself to remember the man whose love had, for a brief moment, burnt away the dark corners of loneliness in that strangely empty life. I tried to push away the flood of memories; a year and a half had passed but I was still haunted by the way Nader had ended our relationship – over Skype by telling me that I was too good for him, that he loved me too much – a reasoning, not surprisingly, I had not been able to follow. A few weeks later an email whose words were seared into my mind – he wanted to tell me himself that he was about to marry his ex. My cheeks burnt again with fury, with self-pity. He had loved me so much that he married someone else ... It would be funny if it wasn't so tragic. If it hadn't happened to me.

An old man shuffled into the pew next to me, smelling of cigarettes and stale urine. I wiped the tears from my face and left.

Just five years ago, I had been on top of the world. At thirty-two, I had landed my dream job as editor of a glossy magazine. I was given a department to manage, new business to win, and within a year, that one magazine had grown to three.

My original dream, though, had been to be a writer. In my twenties, I'd worked for a guidebook publisher, combining writing and travel. I had fun all over the world, rejecting the security my parents had steered me towards – no husband, no mortgage, no business card. Just lots of unsuitable boyfriends and stamps in my passport. And then there was a new millennium; my twenties were behind me and life came to get me. I had been left stranded, homeless and broke after a particularly bad break-up and I needed some stability to get over it, to rebuild my life. The security of magazine work beckoned and I landed the Big Job. My parents made no secret of their relief. Finally I had grown up, I could hear them thinking, was settling down. A mortgage and a husband could only be a matter of time.

That first two fast and furious years had been challenging but exhilarating. I didn't mind the long hours, the breakfast meetings, the late nights, the weekend brainstorms – they kept me busy and I was learning a lot. Then, one evening at a restaurant, after a day of making difficult staffing decisions all day, a waiter asked me if I wanted still or sparkling water, and my mind went blank. I stared at him and to my dinner companion's amazement, I burst into tears.

It may be the modern scourge, but I knew nothing really about stress and its long-term effects, beyond the bragging cry from every corner of our building of 'oh I am so stressed.' After all, stress was the necessary fuel that oiled the wheels of deadlines and high-octane magazine production, an essential by-product of the coalface of creativity we toiled at.

Once stress had moved in, it took over completely. Life was a storm and I was just battling through it every day. Harder to ignore was the weight that started piling on and the spots that erupted. Two years into my job, a few months after a new boss had been put in charge of my department, I was covered in acne. I was already in a daily battle with clothes that pinched and pulled, but with my skin so marked, I could barely face the day. Increasingly, a blank feeling washed over me, and when I wasn't required to deal with urgent situations, my mind fogged over.

I thought I was just tired. But on the first morning of a trip to an exotic resort in the Maldives – one of the perks of my job – I could not get out of bed, waking up crying for no reason, filled with an emptiness that made it impossible to know how to get through the day – even though all it promised was sunshine and the sea – let alone the whole lifetime that stretched ahead of me.

Burn-out. I had lain in that vast bed with its high-thread Egyptian cotton sheets and I thought how appropriate that expression was. I did feel burnt out: emptied of all joy, my energy in cinders, all curiosity in myself, the world and others a pile of ashes.

It didn't help that I was single and my figure did not conform to the emaciated proportions magazines like mine glorified – I myself had fallen victim to the deep dissatisfaction with real bodies that magazines so shame- lessly promote with endless pictures of impossibly skinny young things whose pubescent bodies and youthful skin are retouched to an unattainable perfection that we beat ourselves with. The irony did not escape me.

But here's the curious thing: I wasn't overeating. I wasn't drinking gallons of champagne at every launch and fashion party, stuffing chocolate on the sofa late at night. I had nutritionists and experts coming out of my ears. I had embraced the sweatiest forms of yoga. I had found a healer and experimented with my diet based around the allergies and food intolerances she diagnosed. I gave up smoking and drinking and eating meat. I carried with me a pillbox housing an assortment of vitamins and minerals, tiny bottles of Bach flower remedies and miniature homeopathic pill dispensers. The fridge in the office overran with sheep's milk yoghurt, my usual desk-bound breakfast. I did everything I was told by my experts, embraced every health-food fad going.

Nonetheless the weight kept piling on.

One day, in the thick of this, one of my male friends had bluntly told me that I needed to lower my sights to men of my own 'level of attractiveness', his pointed look at my muffin top telling me how far I had plummeted. In bed that night I had wept hot angry tears, hating myself for caring so much about what he'd said.

At work, the pressure only increased. The size of my department's second-year profits had attracted the attention of management. I had been summoned up to the seventh floor – the executives' floor. We needed an attention-grabbing appointment to bring even more profits for the company, the managing director had told me. I was excited. The appointed new boss with her stilettos and bulging contacts book was a woman I had admired and longed to learn from. But that feeling didn't last. She sowed the seeds of discord and disunity so expertly it took me a while to see what was going on. Divide and conquer – I had been warned by other editors in the building to expect this – she had plenty of past form. But I had proved too innocent for such games. So over the ensuing years, I had allowed myself to be slowly demoted in all but name and eventually had accepted the redundancy she had offered.

I remembered the day I left so clearly. How, in the end, as I walked out of the doors of the building for the last time – the building I had been coming in and out of since I was nineteen, the longest relationship of my life – it had suddenly struck me as the most hilarious thing, that I should be being paid to not come back to work. This life, this job, that had seemed so serious, so very much my *raison d'être*, suddenly felt like nothing at all. My life, when it came down to it, had proved surprisingly easy to put away.

I had no idea how long my redundancy money would last. With no savings and a mountain of credit cards that needed paying off, I took the (irresponsible, according to my mother) decision to use the money to come to Florence instead of sinking it into my debts and starting again with another job. I had calculated that I could make it last a few months if I lived carefully, perhaps a whole year if I lived very frugally. It would be a challenge – my salary had regularly petered out before I reached the end of the month, spent at first on the designer labels my job demanded, and then on expensive diet plans, personal

trainers and sessions with health gurus. I had no firm plans
for Florence; the agreement with Christobel had been for
me to stay for the winter, and then we would see. I had
bought a small notebook in which to assiduously write
down every penny I spent, determined to get a grip on the
art of budgeting while I was here. But anger and bitterness
raged inside me alongside defeat and self-pity, the voice in
my head repeatedly telling me that I had achieved nothing
and would now fail too at being a writer.

The Ponte alle Grazie, the bridge of the graces, mocked its
own plainness with its name. It was simple and undecorated with five concrete arches, defying the dazzling beauty
of the Ponte Vecchio just upriver. Tourists were visible
through the open arches in the middle, the small windows
of the Vasari corridor blinking along the top, catching
the light. During the bombings in the Second World War,
orders not to destroy the 'Old Bridge' had come from
Hitler himself.

I was retracing the taxi's route from last night, attempt-
ing to ground myself. Over the bridge and along a road
with pavements so narrow that every time a bus hurtled
by I had to breathe in sharply to avoid losing a rib. Giant
grey stone slabs made up the walls of the looming buildings, in places revealed through plasterwork that had fallen
away. Enormous arched doorways opened into shops
with bleached wood floors, sparkling vitrines and artfully
arranged clothes, large windows framed by a border of
rough grey stone, some latticed by ancient-looking protruding iron bars.

I reached the Piazza Santa Croce, just as magnificent in the daylight. Standing in the middle of the piazza in a pool of sunshine under a sky that could have been painted by Tiepolo, the puddles from last night's rain reflecting the clouds, I caught the drifting notes of a hand-held harmonium. A new feeling punched its way through my depression: an almost overwhelming desire to dance. To whirl and twirl my way through this vast space, to pirouette, Gene Kelly-style, over to Dante at the far end, to tweak his nose and laugh in his grim face.

Some years ago, on a romantic weekend in Venice arranged by an ex-boyfriend, I had been so moved by beauty that I had burst into tears. It probably wasn't how he had envisioned the weekend going, but I was so overcome by the exquisite city that I practically sobbed at each new discovery: the art, the architecture, the Grand Canal with its gondoliers, the contrast of sweeping piazzas with quiet little bridges stealing over secret canals. Christobel had warned me of Stendhal syndrome, the well-known condition affecting visitors to Florence who actually became ill from a surfeit of beauty, and on packing for Florence I had slipped in plenty of tissues.

And yet, despite the grandeur of the Piazza Santa Croce, the detail on the Ponte Vecchio, the light bouncing off the buildings, and even in spite of my broken heart and defeated soul, I did not feel the urge to shed a tear. Not even when my walk landed me in the middle of the Piazza del Duomo, my mouth falling open yet again at the ornate white edifice of the oversized cathedral. The massive terracotta dome – Brunelleschi's marvel – soared up behind the facade, the

whole building so huge it dwarfed its piazza. The cathedral
felt crowded by the paraphernalia of its own fame: men at
easels drawing caricatures, horse-drawn carriages waiting
for custom, their horses pawing the ground, tour groups
following leaders bearing flags. Tourists teemed all around
it, like Lilliputians pinning down Gulliver, but the Duomo,
ebullient and preposterously vast, refused to cower.

From there, I was led to Sant'Ambrogio's open-air market by the noise. Working my way through deserted back
streets, I shuffled round a drab corner and the scene burst
to life. The market was hemmed in by parked vans and
scooters, pedestrians were weaving through them, some
heading to the market, some heading away, carrying bags
with bunches of flowers and green leaves sticking out of
the top. In the centre stalls, rainbow-coloured produce
collected around an indoor market hall – through the large
open doorways I could see stalls selling cheese, salamis and
hams, bread, and dry goods. Outside, fruit and vegetables
were laid out under a corrugated-iron roof; inside, sacks
of dried beans and chickpeas stood in huddles, bundles
of oregano, packets of dried chillies and herbs lining the
walls, rows of dried and fresh pasta laid out on shelves.

I felt like I had landed in a Technicolor movie set.

I wound my way through the open-air market, tripping
on the little dogs and wheeled trolleys of housewives. I
watched the women as they held lengthy debates with
the stallholders. I stopped at a fruit and veg stall with
strings of chilli peppers hung like a curtain at the back,
and a sign saying: *peperoncino – viagra naturale!* Seeing me
smile, a jovial man with a mop of thick grey hair and round

red cheeks came over. He had a black hat with a bobble pulled over his ears and he was slapping his gloved hands together, regarding me with crinkly eyes. When I reached out to touch a plump red tomato, ribbed and sculpted in segments as if carved, he called out 'oooooh', in a voice that could have carried across mountains. I drew back as if stung. He addressed me in rapid Italian, indicating that I shouldn't touch the goods. Instead he picked up a brown paper bag and filled it with a few of the large ribbed tomatoes, a handful of frizzy lettuce, a deep green courgette, a small bunch of tapering carrots with long bushy tails, a very white round onion and a clove of garlic. Unbidden, he threw in a bunch of broad-leafed basil for good measure. We communicated in a two-hander mime and as I paid, he grinned, slapping his chest and saying: '*Mi chiamo* Antonio!' He stuck out a black-clad hand. I shook it, introducing myself, surprised that his glove was made of cashmere.

'*Piacere*, Kamin,' he looked amused. '*Allora ci vediamo domani!*'

On the corner I paused at a café with small tables outside set with yellow chrysanthemums. A middle-aged man stood sentinel, looking like a garden gnome in spite of his smart blue shirt and the navy apron at his waist. He greeted me in English, opening a wooden door, inviting me in. The interior was just as charming, with wooden wainscoting, framed advertisements from the 1930s hanging on buttercup-coloured walls. The chairs were red plush theatre seats and instead of windows, the front and street side of the café were made of more glass doors, lined with worn wood and closed with stained gilt fittings. The ceiling was a mesh of carved wooded squares, each inlaid with a band of gold, blue and red paint. The friendly gnome explained: 'Is, how you say, Romanesque, from thirteenth century! All windows are from old *ville* around Tuscany.'

The gnome then took my hand and bowed low over it. 'My name is Isidoro,' he said with a flourish, 'and this is Caffè Cibreo, the most beautiful café in Florence. There,' pointing to a restaurant diagonally across the road, 'is Cibreo the famous restaurant. And there,' indicating through the window a large entrance across the other road, 'is Teatro del Sale, a members' club and theatre. We all one family!'

His enthusiasm was infectious. I introduced myself and asked him for a cappuccino to take away. He looked at me with incomprehension.

'Er,' I dipped into the phrasebook in my bag, '*per portare via?*'

He was now installed behind a small curved bar dominated by a huge Gaggia coffee maker at one end and at the other, a glass cabinet displaying small rolls, tiny bite-sized pizzas, glazed croissants and cakes. Behind Isidoro, wooden shelves were crowded with bottles of spirits, a line of silver cocktail makers. He was puzzled. 'But why? You have no moka at home?'

I wanted to drink my coffee as I walked home to San Niccolò, I explained to Isidoro.

He stared for a minute and then started laughing. '*Ma no!*' he exclaimed, wiping tears from his eyes. 'But why so much rush?' I shrugged. He went on: 'But where is the pleasure? How you taste your cappuccino? *Dai*,' he indicated a table by the front windows, 'sit and I bring you. *Così*, you can enjoy.'

I did as he said, and the Gaggia machine gurgled to life. Pleasure – a new concept in my adult coffee-drinking career. I thought back to London and the preternaturally tall cardboard cups of horrible coffee that I carried around with me everywhere. I hadn't passed anyone this morning carrying a cardboard coffee cup. In the land of coffee, I wondered how this was possible. But then, I hadn't seen any coffee-shop chains either. Somehow Florence – at least the parts I had so far discovered – seemed blissfully divorced from modern cities and their globally branded paraphernalia.

Carrying the frothy concoction over, Isidoro declared proudly: 'I make best cappuccino in Firenze! Try, you see!'

He was right. Not too hot, but not lukewarm either, the cappuccino was rich and creamy. 'We use best milk in Tuscany. Good cows!' he said, lingering, asking me where I was from. He clapped his hands excitedly when I told him. 'Ah! *Londra, che bella!* I was once, was beauuutiful!' Then his expression changed to one of pity. 'But vegetables – no taste!' he had commiserated, hanging his head. Then cheering up as he saw my bag of produce: 'But now you taste REAL vegetables!' How amazing could vegetables be, I thought? After all, surely a tomato is just a tomato.

To his continuing enquiries I told him I was trying to write a book, and he let out a low whistle. '*Brava!*' he said, clapping his hands. 'Not just beautiful, but also intelligent!' he exclaimed. 'You stay and you become Fiorentina! You become part of our family!'

I looked out of the window at the tumult of bodies and mopeds on the corner. In the melee a woman with the look of a young Gina Lollobrigida stopped by the moped she was passing and, leaning down, checked her lipstick in its wing mirror, running a finger along her eyebrows. She looked up and spotted me looking at her, and gave me a wink as she sashayed on. I smiled back at her. Maybe I could stay and become part of this funny family of shameless, elegant Florentines.

I raced home excited to taste the produce after Antonio's performance and Isidoro's enthusiasm about Italian vegetables, my depression of the early morning forgotten. I couldn't wait to make lunch. My only other stop was at the bakery opposite: the *forno*, a family concern run by multiple generations, according to Christobel. A cheery girl stood behind the counter, blonde curls bursting free from a white cap. Behind her shelves were filled with freshly baked bread – small oval loaves, large round loaves, long loaves, brown loaves with seeds cracking their crusts, little round rolls and square rolls dusted with flour. In the vitrine there were large square pizzas that were cut into slices, and sheets of thick flat bread shiny with oil and crusted with salt – *schiacciata*, a sort of Tuscan focaccia which, I discovered tasting a small corner, was delicious, crispy and doughy and just oily and salty enough. I struggled through ordering, but she anyway somehow managed to find out my name and where I came from and I somehow managed to learn that she was the baker's youngest daughter and called Monica. All of this without either of us speaking the other's language: I'd never given so much information about myself to so many people in one day without speaking an actual sentence. Monica gave me a small loaf and I carried it upstairs in a paper bag, pausing a couple of times to catch my breath on the way up.

I couldn't remember the last time my vegetables and bread hadn't come packed in polystyrene and plastic. I unloaded my produce into the sink and washed it all thoroughly. Never having been a great cook – or indeed any kind of a cook – all I made was a simple open toasted sandwich – the bruschetta that Antonio had suggested in an entertaining mime. I was so intoxicated by the smell of the tomatoes that I quickly cut them up into round slices, and placed them on the toast. I drizzled on some olive oil, tore up some leaves of basil and scrunched up a few flakes of sea salt.

With the first bite, sunshine exploded in my mouth, sweet tomato flesh made ambrosial by the salt. The oil was peppery and the basil tangy. Each bite was so full of flavour that I actually sighed. Out loud. I made my way through four slices of bread, olive oil running down my chin.

I thought of Iran when we were given deep red tomatoes to eat as snacks after school, holding them in one hand with a salt shaker in the other, biting into them greedily, the taste of that sweetness. Those Italian tomatoes took me back thirty years and they made me happy. A tomato, after all, is not just a tomato, I thought.

Days passed. I was back at the kitchen table, which doubled as my desk. I stared at the document on the screen of my laptop, taunting me with its blankness. I fidgeted in my seat, picking at my nails, chewing at the skin. There was no Internet in the flat and it was a rude awakening. The shock of not being able to surf the net was seismic. There was no email to check, no Facebook to click on to, no pictures of babies of old school friends to check out, no political debates on which to comment.

Instead, I was confronted by the book I had spent years talking about. Not just any book, but the story of my country, of my childhood, of my Iran, which I had fled as a small child with my parents in the violent days of the revolution. After nearly twenty years away, once I had started to travel back to Iran in my twenties, I had regaled my friends with so many tales of my relatives and the history of my country that they had begged me to get it all down on paper instead of making their heads spin with the cast of thousands that makes up my extended family.

But after years of being too busy to think, the shock of having nothing to do but write was astonishing. I gazed out of the window but there was nothing to see: an old lady was at her television in the window opposite mine, the courtyard was quiet, there was just a smell of woodsmoke which floated to me across the city. Inside me, I felt the familiar pull of my old bedfellows, fatigue and depression. So persistent were they in their devotion that nothing I had tried could shake them, not even after nights of sleep so long I felt like Sleeping Beauty's somnambulant sister. *What was I doing here, in this country, a stranger who didn't speak the language and was loved by no one?* Another mistake, I thought, tears welling up, my mother had been right when she had called me irresponsible.

I forced myself to get up, away from the blank document and outside the door, into the streets of Florence, tangible and real. I went out without a map, preferring to wander and discover where I had been afterwards. I paid attention to what was around me instead of peering into a screen all day. My mobile phone couldn't access a network in Florence, so I had no digital way to track my movements. Soon this felt liberating: the ever-present tower of Palazzo Vecchio anchored me, wherever I was in town, I knew that the river and my neighbourhood lay just beyond it, the terraced hills above the Oltrarno the backdrop to my home. And then at a certain juncture in the town, my tower swam into view. It was easy to lose myself knowing that these markers would bring me home.

To my surprise – notwithstanding my British reserve and Londoner's habit of catching no one in the eye – it proved impossible to stay anonymous in San Niccolò. Within days of my arrival, people had started calling out '*ciao*' and giving me a cheery wave when I walked by. And I had returned their greetings – only the horror of being rude beat the horror of being engaged in conversation in the street – and before long I knew my San Niccolò neighbours by name. There was red-haired Cristy. She owned a tiny electrical shop on the street, a middle-aged lady usually surrounded by a tangle of fairy lights, light bulbs and boxes of tiny fuses. Every time I walked past her shop, she professed, in stumbling English, to find me charming.

'*Bella!*' she would exclaim, sweeping her hands around my face. 'So nice, so kind, your smile! Oh yes, *brava!*' and she bobbed up and down, almost bowing in her enthusiasm for my very being.

Opposite Cristy's shop there was a small jewellery shop occupied by another Giuseppe, this one the polar opposite of my neighbour, a gnarled hippie of indeterminate age with long fuzzy colourless hair loosely pulled back into a ponytail. Very short and very rotund, he wore black and smoked roll-up cigarettes, the mongrel at his feet barking as I went by. He introduced his partner, a small woman with dirty-blonde hair who reminded me of a used-up Tilda Swinton, if Swinton had been a foot shorter, smoked 120 Marlboro Red a day for thirty years and not taken care of her teeth.

There were the two sprightly old ladies who I had seen on my first day. They patrolled the street, arms linked, walking the length of San Niccolò, visiting the *forno*, then the greengrocer, then the butcher, until they arrived at Rifrullo for their cappuccinos. They made their stately progress every day, nodding to me, their hairstyles carefully teased into shape, their cheeks always powdered and their lipstick always on.

I had not been able to escape the old man who had joined me in the church that first day. I saw him often on the street and he always smiled at me so hopefully that one day I had paused and let him engage me in conversation. Wheezing, he had spoken to me in surprisingly good English and I had taken pity. He was called Roberto and, after commiserations on the tastelessness of English vegetables, he had placed a hand on my arm, and regarded me intently. 'And who was it who made you so sad?' he asked, catching me by surprise. I reached for the English hauteur I had used all my adult life like a protective cloak, when, looking down at the arthritic fingers clawed around my sleeve, my heart softened. Tears filled my eyes and all my defences fell away.

I had been fighting for so long – the deadlines, the stress, the debacle of my career, and finally, the fight to try to keep Nader's love – and I was exhausted. I gave in, I allowed old Roberto to squeeze my arm, allowed him to comfort me in his creepy way. 'Ah well,' he said quietly. 'No matter, forget him. Now you are in Florence!' He smiled at me kindly, revealing stained teeth. I gave him a watery smile back. 'You are a beautiful woman and you should be in a beautiful place. Stay here and you see, the beauty will make you better!'

I found this encounter oddly moving.

One evening, I went out looking for an Internet café – though a free WiFi line had unexpectedly appeared one day, it switched off promptly at 6 p.m. I tried Rifrullo first, but after dark, it morphed from lively neighbourhood café into one of Florence's trendiest bars. The Rifrullo Pavarotti was replaced by boys with hair gelled into fins, the lights were low and the music was thumping. A crowd of young and beautiful Florentines thronged, both inside and out, regardless of the inclement weather – all Italians, it seemed, smoke – girls with long hair running down their backs like waterfalls, nubile bodies poured into tight jeans; boys with Hoxton mohicans and thick eyebrows in leather jackets and skinny jeans. They were a cross between hipsters and Fellini characters, gorgeous, luscious and voluble. It was no place for me and my laptop.

I walked on to the Piazza Demidoff opposite the river, a wide square with a garden in the centre where smartly dressed locals walked their dogs. At the far end of the square I spotted a small bar with a large sign advertising free Internet. Called the High Bar, it was small and cosy, with wooden booths in the back room. I stepped in. There was no thumping music, only songs that I instantly started to quietly sing along to. The bartender was a small slight man with dark-blond hair and green eyes, his apron tied tight around skinny hips. He smiled.

'*Salve*,' he said and I copied him, using the age-old greeting, the politest way to address a stranger. As a veteran of all of Astrix's adventures, I had to stop myself from raising my arm in a Roman salute.

The High Bar was filled with old-fashioned bar signs and stained antique mirrors and it was empty of other people. Squeezed into a booth with the rain falling outside, I lingered over a mineral water while I skyped with friends to a 1980s soundtrack.

I went there most evenings. One evening, the barman and I found ourselves both singing along to 'Last Christmas'.

'I think we must be around the same sort of age,' I ventured afterwards. 'You play all the music I grew up with.'

'Yes, *bella*,' said the bartender. 'We are. You were born on the eighteenth of September just two weeks after me ...'

I looked at him with alarm. 'How do you know that?'

'Because, Kamin Mohammadi, born in Iran, British citizen, every time you come in here to use the Internet, I have to fill out this book,' he pulled out an A4 notebook filled with dates and times. 'Anti-terrorism laws. So when you come I have to copy out the details of your passport which you gave me first time, and when you came in and how long you stayed online.'

'Good God, poor you!' I cried. 'I do apologise, that must be boring.'

'Well, at least it's something to do,' he said wryly, indicating the empty bar.

'So we are twins?' I smiled, warming to him.

'*Bella*, obviously I am MUCH younger than you!' he threw back with a twinkle.

'By how much?' I demanded. 'A whole year. And you know very well, *cara*, that at our age every day – every second – counts!'

I decided I loved this man.

This was Luigo. He told me his real name was Luigi but the nickname he had acquired from ten years of living in London had stuck. He regaled me with tales of his adventures in London, the dives he had lived in, the fun he had had in the gay clubs, the restaurants he had worked in, how he never got over the awfulness of English food, how when his non-English-speaking mother came to visit him and got lost, she would go into an Italian restaurant brandishing a piece of paper with his address on it and say to the waiters in Italian: 'I am the mother of one of you. This is where I have to go,' and invariably the Italian boys would embrace her and put her in a taxi home.

'She thought London was the friendliest place on earth!' Luigo said with an arched eyebrow. We laughed our heads off.

I looked forward to my nightly visits to the High Bar, not least of all because Luigo introduced me to the concept of *aperitivo*. He forced so many plates of his homemade bar bites on me that I never needed to eat supper when I visited his bar.

This Italian tradition was new to me. Luigo explained that *aperitivo* was dishes of food that were put on the bar and given free to customers to accompany their drinks. 'We Italians never drink without eating,' Luigo said airily. Not for them the pursuit of inebriation as a self-contained leisure activity – 'like in England, *bella*!' he pulled a face. 'Where do you put all that beer? And at lunchtime too! No wonder all those middle-aged men are so fat. Have you seen a man with that belly in Florence?' I had to admit that I had not.

'For us,' said Luigo proudly, 'drinking is always with food and you know we don't count wine as alcohol. For us Tuscans, red wine is food!'

Aperitivo is an early-evening tradition where an after-work or pre-dinner cocktail is taken with plenty of nibbles to stave off any drunkenness. But nibbles did not mean a bowl of stale dry-roasted peanuts. There were full trays of dishes on offer, often a variety of cold pastas and, in Luigo's case, panini cut into tiny squares with different fillings: mozzarella, tomato and basil, prosciutto and rocket, thick slices of mortadella, tuna and cucumber. There were cut vegetables placed next to a bowl of a dressing so delicious I

asked him what was in it. 'Pinzimonio,' he told me proudly.
'It couldn't be easier. You take olive oil – the good stuff of
course – and you mix it with either balsamic vinegar and
salt, or, as I have done tonight, with lots of lemon juice,
some very fine pieces of garlic, and sea salt. Delicious, no?
That way you can eat your celery every day – you know celery is a food of the gods?' I had never been particularly fond
of celery but, dipped in copious amounts of pinzimonio, I
thought I could probably bear to eat it every day.

Every evening I watched him go through the ritual of
putting out the *aperitivo*, placing the trays diligently on the
counter, and then meticulously clean and polish behind
the bar, whizz round lighting candles on each table. One
night I wondered aloud why he bothered with all these
extra touches when so few people came in. He cried out
in protest.

'But *bella*, I do this for me!' he said in mock indignation. 'You see, in Italy, it's important for us to make *la bella
figura* at all times in all things.'

'*La bella figura?*' I echoed. 'The beautiful figure? What,
like being in shape?'

'Er, well no,' he said, pausing in rearranging the bottles
on the shelves behind him, lining up all the labels. 'It's the
principle of making everything look as nice as possible.'

'What, keeping up appearances? Like the Brits do?'

He poured himself a small beer and crossed over to
my side of the counter, guiding me to a table where we
both sat.

'Maybe a little,' he demurred. 'But really, *la bella figura*
is about beauty. You have noticed all the beauty, *si?*' He

swept his hand towards the door, outside which Florence sat lit-up in all her dazzling glory. I nodded. 'Well, beauty is important to us Italians, we revere it. So *la bella figura* is about being the most beautiful you can be, all the time, in every way.'

'Blimey,' I said, 'sounds exhausting.'

'Well, yes, it can be if you're not used to it. But you know it's not just what you wear, or how you look, or keeping your figure slim.' Luigo took a sip of his beer. 'I mean, is also. But it's more about taking care, of speaking beautiful words, being beautiful to yourself, even in private.'

I must have looked puzzled, as he rushed on.

'Look, for example, at home I eat before I come here. I set myself a nice table, put a napkin, maybe a flower on the table, a glass of wine. I cook a good meal, even if is just a quick pasta, salad, *contorni*. Is not because there is someone there to keep up appearance. But for me. I make *la bella figura* for me, because it makes me happy inside. It makes me beautiful,' he framed his face with his hands. 'Is sort of self-respect.'

I thought about the dirt on the windows of the flat, which annoyed me on sunny days. I pictured the piles of books shoved into corners behind the sofas in Christobel's flat, which I ignored with an effort. I thought of the soap scum calcified on the sides of the sink. I recalled how in London I had gobbled sandwiches mindlessly in front of my computer, days of stepping out of my front door without even looking in the mirror, let alone brushing my hair or putting on lipstick. As if reading my mind, Luigo looked me up and down.

'You, *bella*, well, look, I love you …' he started.

'Aha, but …?' I chipped in.

'Well, haven't you got some earrings? Or lip gloss with you?'

'Er, yes, but—'

'No buts, *bella*,' he said sternly. 'Waiting for a party or a man to make you take care of yourself is bullshit. Make *la bella figura* and make it for yourself. Is not hard. You're a clever girl, look around, work it out for yourself.'

With that he gave me a kiss on the cheek and went back to rubbing glasses. I slunk home to start cleaning.

The flat was sparkling. Books no longer exploded out of corners but lined up neatly on dusted shelves. The kitchen surfaces were so clean they shone. The windows twinkled. I had spent days since Luigo's chat scrubbing and wiping, polishing and hoovering, ordering and folding. The flat felt more spacious, harmonious; the plates, cups and glasses back in their rightful places. During this endeavour I found some pretty white handmade china, and a set of white embroidered napkins. There were woven straw placemats and a large cornflower-blue linen cloth, which I spread on the table. Picking out a pretty crocheted doily that I found screwed up in the back of a cupboard, I ironed it out. It looked charming placed on the blue tablecloth. I washed the cotton and lace curtains that hung over the kitchen windows and they emerged so clean that I could finally appreciate the traditional cutwork embroidery. As I rehung them, I saw the old lady opposite at her window, smiling at me approvingly. I smiled back – one house-proud woman to

another – and surveyed the last few days' activity with deep
satisfaction. If I wasn't on the top floor, I would even now
be rushing out with a bucket to scrub my doorstep.

Next, I laid out all my earrings, of which I had a large
collection, on top of the chest in the bedroom. During my
years of weight gain, I couldn't bear to go clothes shopping, so I had poured my energy into costume jewellery.
And impractically beautiful shoes.

I now used the relics of my old life to dress up my scant
wardrobe. On the wall in the back sitting room I found a
rogue hook and on it I hung a pair of beautiful high-heeled,
strappy sandals in silver and metallic turquoise, the only
pair from my collection I had brought with me. The sun
bounced off them and they sent spots of light around the
room. I fished out my favourite lip gloss – clear and shot
through with tiny gold flakes – and put it by the bathroom
mirror, ready to slick on every morning before leaving the
flat. I thought about the two old ladies and their perfectly
groomed appearance on the street every day. I would now
face the day with the same spirit, if with less solid hair.

One luminous day, my neighbour Giuseppe appeared
by my side as I was setting off for my morning walk.
I was surprised. In spite of our physical proximity, we
had never actually acknowledged each other. Now he
introduced himself and, finding we were both going
towards the Ponte Vecchio, Giuseppe suggested we walk
together.

We were on the Lungarno, the road that ran alongside
the river. I was a fast walker, my London pace designed

to cut through anyone who stood between me and my
desk. Giuseppe's walking pace, though, was hesitant
and so reflective of his thoughts that our walk from
San Niccolò to the Ponte Vecchio – which normally
took marching me ten minutes – took us over twenty.
Giuseppe stopped dead every few steps to wave his arms
around and ponder, to scratch his chin and ruminate on
his thoughts. And I, trotting by his side, half his height,
bumped into him or stumbled on the paving stones, surprised by the change in his gait. As we made our awkward progress down the Lungarno, we passed various
red-faced girls jogging, iPods strapped to upper arms,
earphones plugged in, sweat dripping. Giuseppe paused
again with each jogger and sighed, contemplating them.
Finally, as the last Lycra-clad blonde panted past, he
said: 'Ah, American students ... always jogging. What
are they running from?'

He stopped completely then, and I stood helplessly
by his side, waiting. '*Festina lente*,' he said. I looked up
at him blankly. He explained: 'It's Latin. It's a phrase
I have been thinking about for a while. It means something like: in haste, slowness. Probably you will want to
think about that too.'

I chewed this over as we arrived at his bank and said
goodbye. 'In haste, slowness.' It sounded like a Zen koan.
I had noticed that no one here rushed about as I did. I con-
sciously slowed down my pace, learning to look up around
me as I walked.

Then one day I found myself standing in a beam of dif-
fuse winter sunlight, and my patient eyes focused in on

motes of dust dancing in the air, in front of the serene face of a carved Madonna on top of a doorway. I noticed the way the light spilt down in a steep angle over the tall buildings, illuminating half the street, and I stood and did nothing but drink it in. It slowed down the beat of my heart, calming me. There was no need to hurry.

Bruschetta con pomodori

Serves 1 (but can easily be doubled or tripled, or quadrupled for friends, lovers, or parties)

1 slice fresh sourdough bread, made in the traditional way
1 tomato
Best-quality extra-virgin olive oil, for drizzling
Flaky sea salt
Torn basil leaves, for garnish

Toast the sourdough bread. Cut the tomato into fat slices and lay them on top, drizzle with olive oil, and scrunch some flakes of sea salt on top. Garnish with basil and serve.

Pinzimonio

Best-quality extra-virgin olive oil
Best-quality balsamic vinegar
Sea salt and black pepper, to taste
Assorted raw vegetables: peppers, carrots, celery etc, cut in long slices

Pour the olive oil into a small bowl. Add balsamic vinegar – a proportion of 1 tablespoon of vinegar to 4–5 tablespoons of oil. Sprinkle some sea salt, grind in some black pepper and whisk with a fork. Serve with the raw vegetables.

(Note: Instead of balsamic vinegar, you can use red wine vinegar, or squeeze in lots and lots of lemon.)

2

FEBRUARY
La Dolce Vita or how to taste the sweetness of life

Produce in season: fennel
Scent of the city: damp and mossy
Italian moment: shopping at the market
Italian word of the month: *nostrale*

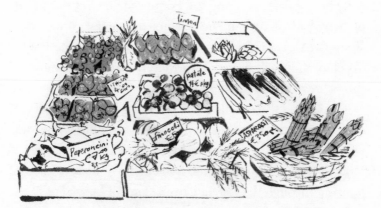

One of the world's most famous museums was fifteen minutes from my flat. The Uffizi was between
my bridge and the Ponte Vecchio on the other side of the
Arno. At the end of the Ponte Vecchio a long loggia of
open arches crawled along the river, its stone legs dupli-
cated in the water. Above the arches was another storey,
punctured with small windows, an unbroken line that
ran from the Uffizi all the way across the river and into
the Oltrarno to the massive complex of the Palazzo Pitti.
The Vasari Corridor had been constructed to allow the
Medici to walk from their palaces on one side of the river
to the other. Giuseppe had told me that there had originally been butchers along the Ponte Vecchio but the smell
of flesh had disturbed the Medici on their promenades
along the Vasari Corridor, and so the edict that the Ponte
Vecchio should house only jewellers had been issued –
this is how it has remained to this day.

The Uffizi palace, unlike the buildings flanking it, jutted
out towards the river, displaying three splendid arches set
with statues and held upright by classical Doric columns –
Vasari's ode to Etruscan classicism. I could see people
pouring through the loggia like an army of busy ants.

I was convinced that Florence was not really a city at all,
but a village. The population was less than half a million,
and while there were some tourists around now, I knew
that the hordes would arrive in the warmer months, when

each Florentine would be outnumbered seven to one by foreigners.

Florence might be a village but a glorious Renaissance village that just happened to produce some of the world's greatest art and architecture, and to invent banking and money in the form of the florin, Europe's first coin. It invented fashion too – an inevitable product of the Florentine love of both art and commerce. Cloth produced from Tuscan sheep had been so brilliantly washed and dyed in the soft waters of the Arno that Renaissance Florence had become the largest cloth-manufacturing centre in Italy. Style and fashion still flows in Florentine veins: Fashion Week was born here in the 1950s, before Milan stole her crown in the 1970s. So a village then, but one that just happened to have people buried in its churches whose names are instantly recognisable: Michelangelo, Galileo, Lorenzo di Medici, Machiavelli, even Lisa Gherardini – the Mona Lisa herself.

Soon after arriving, I had applied for a 'Friend of the Uffizi' card which, for an annual fee, would give me unlimited entrance to all the state museums without having to book or queue. It took me a few days of poking around the Uffizi's large crowded courtyard and colonnaded outer halls to locate the Friends office. The lady in the office gave me an appointment for three weeks later. I asked why I couldn't simply make my application then. She looked at me as if I had asked her to resurrect Michelangelo so I could meet him.

'But no, is not possible now,' she said as if the reasons were obvious. 'You must come back on 1 February.

Opening hours from ten until five, but the office is closed between twelve and four for lunch ...'

The appointed day arrived and the lady grudgingly handed over the card with my name on it. The Uffizi seemed to want to actively discourage people from having easy access and I couldn't really blame it. Outnumbered as they are by tourists, perhaps this was just one of the ways in which Florentines fought back against the mass invasion of their city.

Elated by this victory, I popped into the great gallery, skipping happily past the queue and presenting my card with a flourish, entering the venerable halls with the same thrill as when blagging my way into London nightclubs when I was seventeen. I wandered the famous corridors, walking into rooms arbitrarily, until I was stopped in my tracks by Botticelli's enormous painting of the Birth of Venus, shining down golden from the wall. I sank down on the seat in front of it. I had no desire to go anywhere, just to take in every detail, letting the colours, her expression, the light emanating from the painting seep into every bit of me. The healing power of beauty. Wasn't that what Old Roberto had said – stay and let the beauty heal you?

February had arrived with an extra-cold blast and one day early in the month, I noticed with a shiver that the heating had stopped working. When I met Giuseppe on the street outside the *forno* that morning, he promised to send me Guido, the old plumber who had one of the workshops on the street – San Niccolò was lined by work-shops and artists' studios, old-fashioned even for Florence.

I knew Guido by sight; I saw him every day in Rifrullo talking at the top of his voice to Pavarotti, or on the street shouting out instructions with much gesticulating to his young sidekick. A large round man with white hair and a worn-in face, Guido was a deeply embedded part of San Niccolò life, and now at seven o'clock in the evening he puffed up my stairs tailed by his handsome assistant.

When they rang my doorbell, I was talking to Kicca in London on Skype, the free WiFi having mysteriously failed to switch off as usual. Kicca has been my closest friend since we met in London more than fifteen years ago. Nearly every memory of the past two decades of my life included her – the parties, the boyfriends, the happiness, the tears, the wardrobe crises – she had been there through them all.

Kicca was from Rome, beautiful, black-haired and black-eyed, slim with an athletic figure and a natural six-pack that never ceased to impress me. She had impeccable taste in everything; her dress sense was artistic, colourful and elegant, she cooked beautifully and her homes were always gorgeously eclectic shrines to her travels. Kicca displayed the best example I knew of *bella figura*; way before I had come across the concept, she embodied it.

She had lately discovered another passion: tango. And, irrespective of the fact that she was in her late-thirties and had never had any dance training, Kicca had, of course, in her typical way, started dancing professionally on the London stage within months of starting to take lessons. It wasn't long before her passion drew her to visit Argentina and on her return she told me she had decided to move to Buenos Aires as soon as she could sell her flat in London.

When she announced her decision to leave, I cried for a
month. I could not imagine life without her.

And then I too was suddenly on the move. To Kicca's
home country, no less. Perhaps I rushed off to Florence so
quickly because I couldn't face seeing Kicca leave. In the
end, I left London before she did – Kicca was still busy
preparing her move when I arrived in Florence.

Now, as Guido knocked on the door, I kept the video
on; she could help me communicate with him. I invited
him in, showed him to the kitchen and pointed him to my
laptop, where Kicca's face filled the screen. His eyebrows
shot up when she started to talk to him in Italian and he
chuckled. '*Ma dai!*' he exclaimed. '*Guarda* Gabriele,' indicating the sidekick, '*vieni a guardare ...*'

Gabriele's dark curly hair was worn a little long,
there was an earring in his left ear and muscles rippling
under the wintery layers of clothes. He too peered at
Kicca and they all started talking at once in the Italian
way. Finally, Guido held up an authoritative hand, and
Gabriele fell silent while Kicca explained the problem.
Off they went to the bathroom to examine the boiler,
Guido reappearing after a few minutes. Looking at me,
with a spanner in his hand, he explained something to
Kicca while Gabriele walked through the kitchen and
out of the flat. Kicca translated for me: Gabriele had
been dispatched to the studio to get a spare part that
would fix it. In the meantime, Guido was in the mood to
chat. I offered him a coffee and a chair. He declined the
coffee but sat down gladly in front of Kicca on the computer, leaning into the screen.

He pointed to Kicca's dance partner who was busy preparing dinner in the kitchen behind her and asked if that
was her husband and what he was doing. Kicca was laughing too by now, saying to Guido that no, this was not her
husband, but Guido would not stop.

'*Allora, fidanzato?*' I recognised the word for boyfriend
but as she was trying to explain, he interrupted her, quiz-
zing her on what he was preparing for dinner and for a
few moments they chatted about food, Guido lamenting
Kicca's misfortune at being stuck in 'the land of tasteless
vegetables'. Eventually, she told me that he had finally
approved her dinner and wanted to know what I was eating tonight.

'He says he is worried you don't eat properly, darling,'
she said, still laughing, as he interjected with dramatic gestures from his seat. 'He says you only eat a slice of pizza for
lunch – he's discussed it with Pierguidi the baker ...' At
my protestations, Guido himself addressed me in Italian.
'He wants to know what you are going to cook for dinner?' Kicca translated.

'Tell him I can't cook. I will probably just go to Luigo's
and have some bits and pieces. Or open a tin of tuna ...'

At this Guido grew agitated. He approached my fridge,
and, opening it, he pulled out all the salad leaves I had
there. Filling the sink with water, he threw in handfuls of
different leaves and left them to soak. Then he asked me if
I had pasta and a tin of tomatoes.

I pointed him to the cupboard, asking Kicca: 'What's
he doing?'

'Well, it looks like he is going to cook for you ...'

'Are you serious?'

Guido turned towards us and told me, through Kicca: 'I am going to teach you how to make the most simple and delicious dish of pasta. A beautiful woman like you cannot waste away on tins of tuna! *Mamma mia, che peccato!*'

I wanted to say that I was hardly in danger of wasting away but instead I watched him get busy: he smashed cloves of garlic with one big hand clenched into a fist, telling me to open the tin of tomatoes, talking all the while as Kicca furiously translated. I asked why he didn't use the garlic crush I had found at the back of a drawer – there was no need for Kicca to translate his reaction of horror. When Gabriele returned, I watched them both season and taste the tomato sauce as it simmered, discussing whether it needed more salt or perhaps a pinch more black pepper. The flat was filled with noise and laughter and fizzing smells, suddenly, atmospherically, Italian. Guido instructed me to toast some pieces of bread and, pulling them out of the toaster, he cut a clove of garlic in half and rubbed the fat end over the toast, smearing it with a pungent layer of paste. He then cut up a tomato, crushed it on to the toast leaving traces of pulp, poured on some oil, and sprinkled on some salt.

'*Eccolo*,' he said, kneeling on the floor, holding out the plate towards me with a flourish with one hand while the other hand clutched his heart. We were all laughing so much that only Guido's repeated protestations made me eventually reach for a piece of toast. 'Yum,' said Kicca across the ether, her face distorting as she came closer to her camera. 'Crostini! Typically Tuscan, darling, and oh God I wish you could give me one.'

I understood Kicca's envy as soon as I took a bite. Toast had never tasted so good, so sweet, so garlicky, so delicious. I turned to the grinning Guido and offered him the dish. He delicately picked up a small piece with his rough hand. Gabriele too took a slice and for the first time since they arrived, there was silence as we all crunched and 'aah-hed' our way through the crostini.

At some point, Gabriele went to the bathroom and fixed the boiler while I filled what looked to me like an unnecessarily large pan full of water at Guido's insistence.

'Pasta,' Guido explained, leaning over me, 'needs a lot of water and space to turn in. This is not too big, even for one portion.'

He saw me reach for the oil to pour into the water, and gasped dramatically, holding my arm. 'No no no no!' he admonished. He told me that if the pan was large enough for the pasta to move freely in the water, there was no need for oil to stop it sticking together, just a quick stir when the pasta was first thrown in. He added salt only when the water was boiling. By now Gabriele had joined us in the kitchen, and as Guido and I bent over the stove, I noticed him talking urgently to Kicca, having taken off his jacket, flexing his muscles, striking pose after pose.

'He is asking me if I think he's handsome,' Kicca couldn't stop laughing now. 'Darling, these two are the most dramatic plumbers I have ever met. They make me miss my country!'

Guido snapped curtly at Gabriele and he stopped posing and got busy draining the lettuce leaves and drying them in a tea towel the ends of which he held together and swung around to absorb the water. Throwing the leaves into the bowl I gave him, he dressed the salad with oil, the juice of half a lemon and plenty of salt. He indicated for me to taste – it was delicious, the salad leaves crisp and fresh, the dressing just sour enough. I thanked him and he blushed, placing the salad on the kitchen table. He joined Guido in draining the pasta, the two of them throwing the twists of fusili into the pan of simmering tomato sauce, Guido stirring it all with a wooden spoon to make sure each piece of pasta was coated with tomato, while Gabriele tore leaves of basil into the mixture.

I fetched a plate and set a place. The men handed me the steaming bowl of pasta, the smell filling my kitchen. They pointed for me to sit down, while I kept repeating 'Grazie. Grazie mille!' unable to quite believe what had just happened.

Guido and Gabriele bowed deeply, Guido taking my hand and kissing it. 'Now eat immediately, it's no good cold! We will see ourselves out.'

And with that, the Dramatic Idraulici left me with a home-cooked meal on the table, my radiators fired back to life, and the best laugh Kicca and I had had together in ages.

I decided to try the simple pasta sauce for myself a few nights later. And I managed it OK, by and large, at least after I had put out the fire that flared out of the oil I left on the stove for too long. Throwing in the tomatoes, the flames that exploded from the pan nearly took off my eyebrows. I turned off the heat and flapped at the pan with a tea towel. The fire soon died and, once I had opened all the windows to clear the smoke and wiped up the splattered oil, I managed the rest of the recipe with no further incident, not even overcooking the pasta which Guido had insisted had to be *al dente* – with a bite. I may have had to pencil in part of my singed left eyebrow for a week, but I was proud nonetheless of my first home-cooked Italian dish.

I was standing by Antonio's stall, a still point in a crush of moving bodies at Sant'Ambrogio market, being tutored in the many varieties of tomato. I was now addicted to my bruschetta and *pasta al pomodoro*, and I had come to Antonio seeking some knowledge on my new love. He took me on a journey of discovery: oblong San Marzanoes, the teardrop Roma, small scarlet Pachinoes strung like rubies on the vine, scarlet Datterini miniature plum tomatoes, yellow pear tomatoes like tiny glowing light bulbs. And then there were the ones as large as my hand: round, shiny and fleshy beef tomatoes and the ribbed tomatoes called Cuore di Bue (beef heart) which had first stolen my heart, sometimes shot through with flashes of green. There was even a blue one, which Antonio presented to me with as much pride as if he had grown it himself.

I came here every day, taking home just enough for two days so I could eat as fresh as possible, as Antonio had advised. It was good for me; not just the fresh produce but the walk, the movement, the planning of what I could eat – it helped break up my days and kept the dreaded depression at bay. First of all Antonio had taught me the word '*nostrale*', meaning the produce was local – 'ours' – not flown in from the other side of the world. '*Eh*,' said Antonio, miming an airborne plane, his scarf flapping as he flew around his stall, his arms outstretched, 'I'm dead after fourteen hours on a plane, imagine how the fruit feels!' He snored dramatically. We had developed our own language, a mix of English, Italian and gestures that I instinctively understood. '*Eh*, no!' he wagged his index finger sternly. 'No, food should come from here, *qui*! It is what the land gives you, *la terra*!' he dug with an imaginary shovel. 'The land decides, the season decides, not the aeroplane!' His fingers became snowflakes and he shivered wildly in invisible snow. I laughed, and he laughed too – but I took his point. His wares were grown in local allotments and market gardens on the outskirts of Florence. What Tuscany could not provide was driven up overnight from the south.

Mornings at the market had converted me to the sensual pleasure in the feel, look and smell of a leaf of lettuce so newly out of the ground that it was still speckled with earth, or the beauty of a particularly fat, well-formed fennel, excitement at the arrival of the season's radishes, a blush of magenta on white. It was an excitement that transported me to my grandmother's kitchen in Iran; I could see her now walking in with an armful of radishes, us crunching our way through them with every meal. Antonio quickly laughed me out of my desire for things I couldn't find, such as avocados, telling me I could probably get one in the larger supermarkets, imported from South America. 'But they are sad,' he pulled a long face. 'They suffer, they jetlag!' I was disappointed but mostly because it had taken me so long to figure out how to mime 'avocado' in a way that Antonio would understand.

Not since leaving Iran had fruit and vegetables tasted so good. The Florentines were right: English produce had been a poor substitute. As a child, I had been accustomed to the cornucopia that was typical in Iran. Every home displayed a bowl with so much fruit piled in it that I used to wonder if invisible wires were keeping them in place. Tiny sweet golden grapes, white juicy peaches, small cucumbers we ate cut in halves and sprinkled with salt. The taste memories had never left me – and nor had the shock of arriving in the drab England of 1979 where we queued in the supermarket behind lines of people buying one orange, one apple and one banana each. Fruit in England seemed to mean just those three things. At my boarding school, I had experienced tinned fruit for the first time – things I had been used to eating fresh were now pitiful in syrup so sweet it made my teeth hurt. Although the ensuing two decades had changed the food culture in Britain for the better, I still had not tasted a tomato in London that bore any resemblance to those we had consumed in Iran, biting into them like apples. Now, those taste memories had come flooding back and I couldn't get enough.

Luckily it was all very affordable, as the prices in my notebook showed me. I whiled away whole mornings just enjoying the market: strings of red chillies and bulbs of garlic hanging like charms, bunches of herbs pretty as a bouquet of flowers, the sound of the banter, the colours of the day. On the walk over the river I got to know the streets, the state of the cobbles, the potholes to avoid, inhaling deeply the smells of the city in winter – the faint hint of mossy damp in the narrow streets, a whiff of cologne left in a deserted alley by an Italian man. It rained frequently and I danced my umbrella around other pedestrians on narrow pavements. I ceded them to old Florentine ladies in their furs who would not give way even an inch. It was easier to step off into the street and risk being run down by a bus than try to budge them. They owned their city completely, as immovable as the massive stone walls of the Renaissance palazzi in the centre, with their huge blocks of *pietra forte*, solid and obdurate.

One lunchtime Kicca peered at my groceries across the continent and listened to me rave not just about tomatoes but blood-red oranges too – so dark they were practically purple. She asked me if I had any fennel and when I said yes – the exquisite delicacy of fennel being another new discovery – she told me how to make a ruby orange and fennel salad, a seasonal dish that she herself loved.

I followed her instructions, the oranges staining my fingers red. With two thick slices of Tuscan bread on the side, Kicca also eating her lunch on the screen, I savoured the mix of sweet orange and crunchy aniseed flavours, feeling very pleased with life indeed.

Something curious was happening. My jeans were loose. Used as I was to the monthly vagaries of my waistline – bloating with certain foods, swelling with the monthly cycle – I took no notice at first. But it persisted until there was no ignoring it.

I had spent most of my life on a diet. But here in Florence, I had given myself permission to stop counting calories. In fact, I had been committing the ultimate sin: living on carbs, sleeping with (or rather devouring) the enemy. Dr Atkins would be spinning in his carb-free grave.

For the first time in years, I was revelling in food. And much as I awaited my punishment, all this joyous indulgence was having the opposite effect. It was all the walking, I decided: each evening I climbed the steep steps up behind San Niccolò to watch the sun set over the city and as I went up and down the four flights of stairs to the flat several times a day, I no longer puffed or had to stop to rest halfway up. I was exercising more than when I used to force myself to go to the gym, feeling out of place as all around me muscle-bound types in tight Lycra gazed at their own reflection doing bicep curls, worshipping intently at the temple to the body beautiful.

But what if it wasn't just the walking and the stairs? I looked around my kitchen and it struck me with the clearness of San Niccolò's church bells – everything I was eating was fresh and natural.

In London, I had existed on pre-packaged 'health' foods, full of ingredients so adulterated they bore no relation to their original state, filled with preservatives and additives, packed in enough cellophane and plastic and cardboard to build a shanty town. I had had no time or energy to cook for myself.

Now I carried a large straw bag I'd found in the cupboard
to the market every morning and Antonio filled it with
fruit and veg, no plastic bags or useless packaging needed.
I snacked on fruit and vegetables (and daily celery) instead
of power bars or sugar-free gluten-free biscuits for no other
reason than pure taste sensation. And pleasure. The concept
that was so alien when Isidoro had talked of it in my first
week in Florence had become my main motivation.

From the earliest age I had learnt to think of myself
as fat. I had been a chubby child and my mother, who I
have never known not to be dieting, preferred to feed
me instead of herself. It was her way of showing love and
I, wanting to please her, had eaten it all up. I remember her denying herself the delicious fare that she heaped
on to our plates: she was the hostess and her slim figure
was important. She had always been keen on exercise, and
in the 1980s she had followed the Jane Fonda aerobics
craze. I made my friends laugh by ridiculing Fonda's calls
to 'go for the burn!' but I pinched what I thought was fat
around my waist and did Jane Fonda's workouts in secret.
Although we did enough sports at school to keep us in
good shape, as we journeyed through our teens, we all
competed for who could hate their body more. The only
thing we didn't learn was how to be satisfied with ourselves, to see the dazzling beauty of our young skin and
firm high breasts. Looking back at photos of myself at the
age of seventeen, I see a perky young woman with luscious curves and great legs. But at the time all I could
see was a body that did not resemble in any way that of
Christie Brinkley or Cindy Crawford.

When I had binged on beer in my first year at university and, happily in love with my first serious boyfriend, also gorged on takeaways, I really did start to get fat. Following my mother's lead, I went on a diet. I discovered iron self-discipline – I had been trained by the best after all – and started to see the pounds fall away. After two weeks I was so delighted that I stayed on the diet for three months and added a gym routine to the mix. When my hip bones were jutting and my eyes were twice their size in my sculpted face, my mother finally regarded me with approval, and took me out shopping to buy a whole new wardrobe of skin-tight clothes.

By the time I had landed my editorship in my early thirties, I was a happy size 8 who probably drank and smoked more than I ate, but I was so proud of my slim figure I didn't care what it took to maintain it. Once the weight started piling on, I pursued all the diet fads going – the Hay Diet, the Dukan Diet, the cabbage soup diet, the grapefruit diet, the blood type diet, the maple syrup diet, even the baby food diet. When none of those worked – I had regular dizzy spells at my desk like some nineteenth-century heroine from Russian literature – I turned to nutritionists and alternative health, trying out allergy tests, this time eliminating 'bad' foods. I gave up sugar, wheat, gluten and yeast. I gave up whatever that month's nutritionist or diet book told me to give up. When I had so restricted my diet that even bananas were out of the question, I took to my bed for a whole weekend until Kicca let herself in with her key and cooked me up a plate of gluten-free corn pasta which, despite her best efforts, tasted like glue. It was Kicca's love and concern that really fed me that dark weekend and coaxed me up and out to face another week.

In stark contrast, I was now surrounded by abundance. A small notice in the bakery said *lievitazione naturale*, which, Kicca explained, meant that they didn't use yeast but a natural raising agent, a centuries-old Tuscan bread-making practice – a traditional sourdough. In London bread had been my enemy. The indigestible 'health' loaves – wheat-free, taste-free – I had chosen, the shelves of bread I had seen in American supermarkets on business trips, every single one of which contained added sugar, the white sliced loaves which turned into paste in my mouth. In London, artisan breads and traditional methods had to be marketed and turned into a movement headed by a celebrity chef. Here, it was just part of the fabric of daily life. This Tuscan bread, made as it was from clean traditional ingredients, did not paralyse my gut with spasms or bloat me so much I looked five months pregnant. It simply nourished me.

In Florence, bread returned to its essential life-giving self.

On one of those misty days when Florence wrapped clouds tight around herself like a stole, I was coming home from the market when I saw Old Roberto on the street corner. I took a deep breath and crossed over. The mist was icy, and the damp felt like it was seeping into my bones.

'You look tired today,' he said, his rheumy eyes raking my face.

Usually when people tell you that, what they mean is 'you look terrible' or 'you look old'. Whichever way you read it, 'you look tired' is never a compliment.

'Huh, well, I slept ten hours last night ...'

'Ah,' he said, 'that's the problem. Too much sleep. It's not good for you. Too much alone in bed.'

I blinked at him, dumbfounded. It seemed unthinkable that he could be making some kind of advance – surely he was over a hundred? Perhaps he was showing grandfatherly concern. Misplaced but well-meaning.

I excused myself, beating a very English retreat up to the nest.

Was it possible that Old Roberto believed me somehow nearer his age than I was? As was becoming usual when I had a dilemma for which I needed the advice of a good girlfriend, I rushed down to Luigo's.

'You don't look a day over thirty-seven, *bella mia* ...' Luigo grinned at me, winking. For the second time that day, I blinked at an Italian man in dismay.

'*Bella*,' he pronounced, 'at a certain age, a woman has to choose between her arse and her face. OK,' as I gasped at this pithy truth, 'don't be too impressed, I know it sounds like one of Luigo's gems, but Catherine Deneuve beat me to it.'

'Define a certain age?' I asked defiantly. Luigo ignored me, dipping a little bread into a saucer of olive oil, soaking it thoroughly and popping it into my mouth.

'Now, take your medicine like a good girl. At least four times a day. Olive oil is the secret of youthful skin. You should see my mother ...'

'But Luigo, I can't go round drinking *oil*! I just lost a bit of weight ...' I protested.

'Oh, shut up with your calorie-counting Anglo-Saxon *cazzate*,' Luigo was stern. 'Now, go and look it up on your

beloved Internet – you are the journalist. I have customers
to attend to.' And with that I was dismissed.

I did go and look it up. And I found out that extra-virgin olive oil is full of antioxidants such as vitamin E (hence
the great skin Luigo had mentioned), carotenoids (the colourful plant pigment which the body turns into vitamin
A) and oleuropein – the enemy of free radicals. I already
knew that antioxidants were the holy grail of health foods,
able to capture and destroy those pesky free radicals who,
I'd always imagined, raced around one's body like a malign
Che Guevara, blowing up collagen bridges and causing
general ageing chaos. I just didn't know olive oil contained
so many of them. It was also packed to the rafters with
monounsaturated fat – the most sought-after of 'good fats'
– which lowers cholesterol and controls insulin, avoiding
the sugar highs and lows caused by spikes in the hormone.
I also unearthed research which suggested that consum-
ing more than four tablespoons a day of extra-virgin olive
oil could lower the risk of having a heart attack, suffering
from a stroke or dying of heart disease, as well as protecting against a bunch of different cancers and delaying the
onset of Alzheimer's.

My research introduced me to the Mediterranean diet
with its cornucopia of fresh vegetables, oodles of olive oil
and even regular shots of coffee, and all the statistics that
backed up its health-giving benefits. Tomatoes, I learnt,
increased their lycopene (a cancer-fighting antioxidant)
when cooked, and especially when combined with the
good fats contained in olive oil. So even a tin of tomatoes combined with pasta – as I did in making Guido's

pasta dish – was filling me with good health. Coffee, I discovered, contains more than twice the amount of heart-friendly polyphenols than virtuous green tea. Good skin and less chance of getting sick? It was a no-brainer. I was converted.

I asked Antonio's advice the next morning at the market. Good olive oil, it turned out, was his favourite subject – after the goodness of tomatoes and the importance of fresh seasonal food. '*La qualità non ha un prezzo!*' he said decisively.

I made a sad face, pulling out the insides of my coat pockets.

'Pah!' Antonio wagged his finger. 'No problem. *Devi semplicemente comprare meno!*'

I had already heard Antonio's thoughts on the importance of quality so I understood that he was insisting I buy less rather than inferior quality. He wrote down an address on a scrap of paper with a stub of pencil he fished from his pocket (and actually spat on the nib, much to my delight), and sent me off. I bumped into Giuseppe en route, ambling towards the market. He examined the paper as if it contained the secrets of life, and eventually said: 'Ah Pegna, yes, a very good place. And Kamin,' he stopped me as I made off, 'they have some unusual cleaning products you will probably want.'

I set off, laughing quietly at the thought that Giuseppe spied on me as keenly – and discreetly – as I did on him.

I dodged into the streets behind the Duomo where I discovered Pegna, the sort of old-fashioned emporium that I've always found irresistible. It stocked everything from the cleaning products that Giuseppe had mentioned to shockingly expensive tins of very yellow butter. It seemed populated solely by fierce old Florentine ladies wearing furs that fell down to their ankles. Short and squat, their hair set, their coats wrapped tightly around them, they were more stoic than glamorous. As I browsed the shelves, their trolleys clipped my ankles, their profiles set as hard as their hair as they swooshed past without a glance.

The whole experience was intimidating – not to mention bruising for the legs – but I located the olive oil Antonio had recommended, winced at the price, swapped it for a smaller bottle and picked up a few other things – excitingly efficient cleaning unguents and a bag of dark chocolate-covered figs it would have been rude to ignore – and headed to the two tills at the front of the shop to pay. At one was parked an old lady as scary as her customers and, at the other, a young woman with a sad Renaissance face and large lugubrious eyes. I chose her till and lined up behind the fur-clad ladies. The radio was on and Amy Winehouse's 'Back to Black' was playing. This song had been the soundtrack to my heartbreak after Nader left me and I knew all the words. The girl at the checkout was surreptitiously singing along under her breath. I was too, an automatic and unconscious response which has, over the years, irritated colleagues no end. For one heartbeat, our eyes locked. Then she sang the next line a little more loudly and looked up at me, a challenge in her eyes. I sang the next line and looked back at her, raising an eyebrow. She took up the next line, her eyes never leaving mine, and so it went on, a kind of singing duel until finally, we duetted through the chorus in full voice as I swept up my shopping bags and left, waving to each other through the window, having not exchanged a word. A few weeks in Florence and I felt like I was living in a musical. Which was how I have always thought life should be. I caught sight of my reflection in a shop window as I walked away. I stopped – for a moment I didn't quite recognise myself. I searched my reflection for changes: all that looking up had improved my posture and my sparkly earrings added style to my black coat and boots, my lip gloss was shining ... but it wasn't just that. I was wearing an expression that it took me a while to place.

I looked happy.

I obeyed Luigo and took my medicine four times a day, like a good girl, sometimes just drinking the olive oil straight from a tablespoon. Drinking the oil neat made me appreciate the value of Antonio's mantra: invest in good quality. He had taught me how to identify good oil by shaking it and judging its viscosity, the amount of bubbles it made in the bottle. I peered at the colour – was it golden or was it greenish – learning that the greener Tuscan oil was fresher and contained even more chlorophyll and antioxidants than the golden oil. It was still only February and the 'new oil' was harvested in late October or early November, Antonio had told me, and still considered fresh for a year. The bitterness to its tang stimulated my taste buds and its, well, oiliness promoted good gut health, something my stressed-out intestines apparently appreciated. Soon, though, I was not taking my oil just as medicine, but enjoying it, learning to love the subtleties in its oleaginous flavour.

Within ten days my cheeks were fuller and there was a different feel to my skin. Plumper, brighter, it had lost the sallowness from years of working in a neon-lit office, a certain grainy quality that no amount of facials had been able to shift. Even better, the last traces of the acne had disappeared, as if retouched by an expert graphic designer. The spots themselves had magically left within weeks of leaving work but some scars had remained and I had gotten used to not looking too closely in the mirror. Now, looking in the mirror was no longer upsetting; I could peer at myself under the brightest light and saw none of the previous marks or lines. Just firm, glowing skin.

And that wasn't all. My eyes now shone and my hair was glossy. The dullness that had settled over me was being sloughed away, from the inside out. My rambling explorations of the city had added colour to my cheeks, brought some much-needed oxygen to my cells; sometimes as I returned from these epic walks and swallowed my extra-virgin cold-pressed green olive oil, I was sure I could feel every cell in my body singing with vitality, vibrating with energy.

That evening, I paid my first visit to San Miniato, the church that sat on the hill above the flat, its marble façade etched on the horizon. The glinting gold mosaic at the top had been my guide home more than once, crowning the terraces that rose up behind San Niccolò. Although I walked up in the hills often, I had never gone in, prioritising the art of Michelangelo, of Giotto, of Boccaccio instead of the little Romanesque church so close to home which held the relics of Florence's patron saint.

I slowly climbed the central staircase, which led to the church. Halfway up, I lifted my face to take in the marble facade, as every bride who climbs these stairs on her wedding day must do. I fantasised that Nader was waiting for me inside that church and I swallowed down the lump that rose in my throat. Would this sadness never end? It had been more than a year now since he had married, surely I should be over him. But now that I was living a leisurely life, the protective barrier of the hectic routine of my former life gone, his memory had returned to haunt me, and I could not put the image of him from my mind.

I stood in the broad terrace in front of the church. San Miniato presented a superlative view over the city. I sat on the wall above the church's cemetery, gazing at the sunset which was putting on a spectacular show of colour and light. I hardly saw this, I was so lost in thoughts of Nader.

We had met in the Napa Valley five years earlier, and it hadn't taken long to make the connection of our shared past – before the revolution, we had attended the same school in Iran. We had stayed in touch and over the years, we had met every time we found ourselves in the same city. He had taken me out for a drink when he had passed through London for business, I had seen him in Washington DC while there on a magazine trip, we had driven in his convertible green Mustang through Tehran when I had been visiting family, speeding along the highways as everyone pointed as if we were famous. Our meetings, always in some different part of the world, were a metaphor for the shifting spaces that we both occupied as uprooted Iranians.

The last time I had seen him had been at a conference in New York when the chemistry between us was so electric that our fellow delegates instinctively cleared a space around us when we all went out dancing on the Saturday night. And yet nothing had happened. After we had bid farewell, a mutual friend had told me that he had a long-term girlfriend in Tehran.

And then suddenly, months later, a brief Skype conversation full of flirtation, and a few days after that I was watching him lug his suitcases up the staircase to my flat. He was bent double, one suitcase lying across his back, reminding me of the old porters in the bazaars of Iran. He dropped his bags in my flat's tiny entrance and we smiled politely at each other across the small space. 'You see,' he said, 'I came. You shouldn't have offered ... you are too polite for your own good, Kamin-*jaan*.'

I had laughed and disclaimed. But it was true in a way – I had not really thought he would take me up on my impulsive offer to visit London. He had put down his bags and taken me out for dinner. In the balmy Hampstead night, we sat out on a restaurant terrace to eat. He had told me then the reason for his unexpected visit, how he had had to leave Iran suddenly for his own safety, how he had landed in Dubai with no plans and no ideas for the future – his life wiped clean with one flight. That was when he had skyped me and jumped at my invitation.

It was not the first time that our country had broken our hearts. Once before, as children, our lives had been wiped

clean with a flight out of Iran. And now it had broken
his heart again, forcing him to flee the life he had reconstructed so painstakingly as an adult, fulfilling his dream
– all of our dreams – to call Iran his home again. We talked
late into the night, wandering the leafy streets after dinner. Somewhere in that conversation he told me that he
was no longer with his girlfriend, whom he had left behind
in Iran. He was free, single at last. With that we had gone
back to my flat, and the sofa bed had remained unmade.

For three months we had shared everything. My little
flat, my cat, my hours off – a life. I had a reason to finish
work on time: I didn't care if I didn't get through that
day's to-do list – at 5.30 I was racing out of the building and back to Hampstead where Nader was waiting for
me, the long light evenings our playground to be tumbled
through together. Over those days, which turned into
weeks, which turned into months, we fell in love. As if it
was always meant to be that way. Nader was the first lover
who understood both my identities, who could laugh at
Western jokes and sing along to Persian songs with me.
He had completed me, and I had fallen into him with total
abandon. I was convinced he would be my husband.

The fiery shades of the sunset roused me. I went into the
church. A beamed and gaily painted Romanesque ceiling
stretched above a marvel of marble: worn marble on the
floors, an intricately carved marble pulpit, slabs of marble delicately inlaid with more marble on the walls. I ran
my hands along their cool grooved surfaces. I had found
plenty of Islamic undertones to the loggias, perfectly
spaced-out arches and inner courtyards in Florence. Every

tour guide I overheard lectured about the neoclassicism of
the Renaissance, the genius of Brunelleschi in copying the
Romans, the Etruscans, the Greeks, but I could see reflec-
tions of uncredited Islamic influence everywhere, and here
in San Miniato, the pattern in the marble, the inlay work,
the motifs used all came from the perfect geometry of
Islamic art. The sound of monks singing vespers pulled me
down to the crypt, their thick robes falling around them
as they chanted in Latin. The ceiling here was low, arched;
there were fat, squat columns. I sat and the sacred music
vibrated through me, here in this womb-like room, protected, at home in that Florentine crypt bearing motifs of
the Middle East.

When the monks had finished their chanting, lit their
candles, and processed out, their rough robes scratching
on the stone floor, I went to explore the church. Up some
stairs I was confronted by a huge mosaic Christ built into
a demi-dome. A small old monk came out of the shadows,
pointing to a sort of slot machine that asked for a euro
to light up the wall. I rifled through my bag but couldn't
find a euro. The old man paused, reaching into the folds of
his robes, and pulled out a coin, pushing it into the slot,
and pointed up to the flood of light that illuminated the
mural. The gold mosaics shone brilliantly and, in the middle, Christ stared at me with Byzantine eyes, dark brown
and soulful. The eyes of the men of the Middle East. The
eyes of my people. The eyes of Nader.

I stared until the time ran out and the light clicked off.
In the sudden dark, I stepped, confused, through a doorway, entering an empty square room lined by carved

wooden choir seats, throbbing with stillness. I sat in the corner, leaning back, hiding in the hard wooden seat, looking at the four frescoes that covered the walls, the two tiny stained-glass windows at the top, feeling breathless, my heart racing. My eyes fell on an angel in the stained glass; it appeared to be radiating light. The stillness around me deepened until it was broken by a deep choking noise. I realised, with detachment, that the noise was a sob and it was coming from me. And then I sobbed violently, my body convulsed.

All the pain poured out: the pain of losing Nader who was my animus, the male me, the one who understood because he had lived the same story. I felt again the agony of his desertion, of his choosing to go back and marry the old girlfriend, the humiliation of being made a footnote, our beautiful romance just a parenthesis to the real story, their story. To be turned into just an affair, an aberration. I howled for the offence to my soul, the blow dealt to my dignity. I felt all the betrayals of the last few years: the duplicity of the Big Boss, the disappointment of my career, the treachery of my body. I don't know how long I was there but eventually I looked up and saw the angel, and it looked as if it was smiling down at me, still mysteriously illuminated, and my cries died down, and, finally, exhausted, I sat there, spent, a deep peace washing through me.

In that moment, I forgave Nader. For playing with my heart and for being careless with it. I forgave it all and I forgave myself too for being so angry, so hurt. Suddenly it felt OK to have had that love; it had been so sweet, so poignant. For those brief months, I had felt understood and contextualised by someone just like me. Someone I didn't need to explain myself to, to spell out the names of my relations, to explain the courtesies of Iranian culture. Someone who understood it all because he was made of it just as I was.

Eventually I left the sacristy and the church. It was now dark outside, and walking down the winding road back to San Niccolò, I felt so light that I started to run and skip all the way home.

The next day, I woke up happy – pointlessly, mindlessly happy. After breakfast (supplemented with a shot of oil), I dressed in the brightest colours I could find and donned the sparkliest earrings I had. At Rifrullo I threw a cheery '*Ciao*' at Pavarotti, taking a seat at my usual table. My cappuccino appeared, delivered with a snatch of 'Nessun Dorma'. As I smiled at Pavarotti, the vegetable delivery man walked by as usual, pushing his trolley past my table. As he did every morning, he looked at me and nodded and as usual I looked back at him and said '*ciao*'. I gave him a smile – that was usual too – but what was not usual was that he looked at me for so long that he crashed his trolley noisily into the next table.

Vegetables tumbled everywhere, potatoes thudding to the floor, onions shedding skins as they spun under tables. He scrabbled around picking up his wares; Pavarotti came out from behind the bar to help, raising an eyebrow fractionally my way. I wasn't sure what had just happened but I knew that there was something different about today. Something had changed; *I* had changed.

About ten minutes later, as he wheeled his empty trolley back through the bar from the kitchen, the vegetable delivery man tossed a folded-up napkin on to my table. And then he was gone.

I picked up the red napkin and unfolded it. Written in a bubbly hand it said:

'*Ti piacerebbe di vederci una sera? Ti lascio il mio numero 335 777 2364.*'

I didn't understand the words, but I got the message. I folded it up and slipped it into my pocket to show Luigo later.

That wasn't the only weird thing that happened that day. On my way to the market, crossing the bridge, I smiled at a man on a moped and he smiled back so enthusiastically that he wobbled dangerously and narrowly missed a bus.

Later, sitting as usual in Cibreo, I saw a new face arriving for work – the manager, Beppe, back from his holidays, tall and good-looking with jet-black hair, and a suit so sharp I could have cut myself on its lapels. As he passed me, he did a double take. And I smiled at him broadly, drinking in his tall, dark and handsome form. He smiled too, looking at me so intently that he tripped over, nearly falling as he entered the bar.

I couldn't ignore this any longer. Once may have been an accident, twice a coincidence, but three men falling over after seeing me smile – surely this was a hallucination? I looked around dumbly for a candid camera, waiting for someone to jump out of the bushes and tell me that it had all been an elaborate joke, or to discover that my morning coffee had been laced with LSD by the Rifrullo

Pavarotti. I had been invisible to men for the best part of the past decade – with the exception of Nader – and after the last disastrous relationship many years before him – with a well-soaked writer who I had left after a year of him repeatedly cheating. Until then, I had been practically celibate, years could pass – had, indeed, passed – without me touching another human being with desire. Typical of publishing, my workplace largely comprised women. With the exception of the genial double act of the two elderly ex-army boys on reception, and the guy who ran the staff café – despite an astonishing lack of aptitude, a man capable of burning even coffee – most of the other men that worked on magazines were gay.

I had had high hopes for Italy. My first experience of the country had been a working trip to Sicily with Kicca. There the men were so intensely predatory that if you caught an eye, he would follow you all night. At times it got wearing and a little worrying. But after a month of this, when I got back to London, I felt bereft. When I walked past a group of workmen and not even one of them raised their head, I confided in Kicca that I missed the attention of Sicilian men. Kicca had laughed: 'Imagine what it was like to move to London aged twenty-five, having grown up like that. No one looked at me. I felt ugly.' She told me that in the first year after arriving in London she had taken to eating Mars bars for consolation, put on two stone in weight, and become depressed.

I went back home and peered at myself in the mirror, looking for an answer. Were my pupils dilated? Was I, in fact, tripping? But my eyes looked normal, if bright. I could see nothing that might signal such a dramatic reaction.

Later, Luigo listened to me carefully from behind the bar. I explained how this sort of thing never happened to me. 'For years I have hardly dated at all. Apart from Nader' – who I'd already told him about – 'no boyfriends or regular dates. There was a famous actor once who I thought was interested ...'

Luigo clapped his hands together when I named the old man. 'Oh, I love him. Those eyes ...'

'I know, but by the time I met him, he was about a hundred.' I paused. 'OK, more like sixty-five, but anyway, old enough to sag. I went to interview him for my magazine and he rang me every time he was in London.'

Luigo gasped with delight.

'I know,' I nodded. 'I felt like that too. But actually, he was launching a new health-food line and I guess he wanted me to promote it. I was such a fool, I actually thought he might want fat, spotty me! This man who had dated the most beautiful women in the world ...'

Luigo tutted at my description of myself, wagging a finger in my face, but I went on.

'Well, once he turned up at the office on Valentine's Day. I was across town on a shoot so I missed him. But everyone in the office saw him, which, let's face it, is almost as good.'

Luigo nodded his agreement.

'I was so excited when I came back – he had left me a note and a package – it was heavy too.'

'A ring with a diamond bigger than Liz Taylor's?' gasped Luigo.

'No, sadly. It turned out to be a loaf of bread ...'

Luigo sat down, deflated. 'Bread?'

'I know,' I said. 'And not just bread, but some proto-type of a gluten-free, wheat-free, everything-free bullshit loaf of bullshit bread. The note was a recipe for goddamn cheese on toast. He called it something posh but that was basically it.'

'And was it delicious?' Luigo couldn't help being Italian.

'What do you think?'

'No? How rude!' For Luigo – an Italian – this was the worst part.

'And get this, that night I had to go out with my staff. They all had their husbands and boyfriends with them. I had my preternaturally heavy loaf of taste-free bread. It sat next to me on the sofa all night. That's the nearest I got to dating. A night out with celebrity bread ...'

When I finished he declared with a flourish: 'So now you see what it is to be a beautiful woman in Italy, *bella*?'

'But I am not beautiful,' I protested. 'And certainly no more than yesterday. Why didn't this happen before? Is it the olive oil?'

'*Bella*,' he said fondly. 'Look at you, how different you are now from when you first came in here. Then you crawled in like a worm, all hunched up and looking at the floor, you said sorry a hundred times. Now ... well, now you bounce in here, head up, walking tall and you look me straight in the eye. No more worm! And when you smile, it comes straight from your heart. You see, now you know the secret to being admired in Italy. It's because you are making *la bella figura*. And let me warn you, Englishwoman, this makes you much more powerful than you could possibly imagine.'

I got an intimation of this power every day when I went to Cibreo with groceries and Beppe took them from me at the door and ushered me in while Isidoro made my cappuccino – I felt like their queen. I sat in the corner, which commanded the best view of the café for people-watching and, more importantly, the bar itself where I could see Beppe as he greeted his customers by name, bending low over the hand of an old lady as he led her to a table and conjured up a glass of water for her to sip. Beppe was charming, solicitous, and beautifully dressed – I was making a study of his suits; there was the sleek navy one with double pockets, the charcoal wool with its gorgeous pile, the pin-stripe with the wide lapels … Each cut perfectly, each one an ode to the stylishness of Italian men.

I longed for him to ask me out. Luigo urged me to ask him instead. 'You are a modern woman!' he said, and pointing out that Beppe was short for Giuseppe, Italian for Joseph, he worked himself up to his joke with a satisfied grin, 'and just because there are many Josephs in your life, *bella*, it doesn't mean you have to be like the Madonna, a virgin! And you know that tomorrow is San Bloody Valentino – why don't you give Eros a hand?'

The evening of San Bloody Valentino, I took Luigo's advice and went to Cibreo at night for the first time. It glowed warm in the chilly night. It was still too early for courting couples; there were just a couple of regulars at the bar, drinking prosecco. I took a deep breath and went in. Beppe was looking more handsome than usual, his dark suit paired with a silk pocket-handkerchief and matching tie. He bounded over to the door to lead me to the bar, pouring me a glass of prosecco and thrusting it in my hand. He then presented me with two small plates. One bore twists and turns of something pickled with strips of onions, carrot and garlic and the other was a golden gloop. He ground some salt and black pepper, poured a little oil over the top. '*Mangia*,' he ordered, 'they are some of our chef's specialities.' Beppe pointed to the pickled one first and I picked up a forkful, biting into it gingerly, but the taste was enchanting. I ate it all up. The other plate was 'polenta with just a little Parmigiano and seasoning,' explained Beppe. He watched me as I cleared both plates, offering me another glass of prosecco. I refused; the place was starting to fill with people, it was time to go home.

He accompanied me to the door. 'Tell me,' I asked him, 'what was the other dish that I tried?'

'The most typical dish of Florence,' he said with a grin. '*Trippa fiorentina*. Tripe!'

I had been a vegetarian for the past fifteen years, only recently starting to eat meat again. I screwed up my face. And that's when he kissed me. His lips landed gently on mine and, for the long seconds that it lasted, it took my breath away.

I walked away stunned. He returned to the bar, gold sparkles from my lip gloss twinkling around his mouth. As I walked past Dante's statue, I found myself licking my lips.

A whole week after the kiss, Beppe finally asked me to dinner. In a move suggested by Luigo, I had invested in some tight trousers to show off the new firmness of my thighs, toned by my walks and the never-ending stairs. Every day at Cibreo, I took off my coat and handed it to Beppe to make sure he noticed. Eventually he must have as he suggested pizza and we fixed a date for Sunday night.

On the appointed day I was dressed, made up and ready in the kitchen early, tapping my fingers nervously on the table. There were fresh sheets on the double sofa bed which I had unfolded, and, for the first time in weeks, I had shaved my legs. In London I had spent a small fortune on going to the woman known for inventing the Brazilian. In a reversal of fortune told through depilation, I had bought wax strips after losing my job but now, with no income in sight, I had resorted to shaving.

When the doorbell rang, I practically ran downstairs to find Beppe slapping his hands together on the doorstep, devastating in a black leather jacket with a black cashmere scarf knotted loosely around his neck. He took my hand and we walked down the street to the local pizzeria where we slid into a booth and barely noticed the delicious pizza. Afterwards, he led me back to my flat, and kissed me the moment we were inside, and didn't stop.

Some time near dawn he left and I fell into a long and satisfied sleep.

'I can see from that glow, *bella*, that celebrations are in order!' Luigo said when he got to work the next evening to find me waiting for him. He poured us both prosecco and clinked his flute to mine. 'Good, I am guessing?'

'Oh my God! Put it this way, afterwards I asked him if he went to circus school ...'

'Cirque du Soleil?' quipped Luigo.

'More like Sex du Soleil!' I said, and we threw our heads back and laughed, high-fiving over the bar.

'You are living *la dolce vita*!'

'I am?' I looked round for paparazzi. 'But I haven't been to any glamorous parties and I haven't swum in a single fountain!'

'*La dolce vita* has nothing to do with Fellini or that Swedish bird with her big tits,' Luigo's mouth curled with distaste. From the sounds of it, Luigo's time in London must have been largely spent with some unre-constructed barrow boys. 'Once we had the might of the Roman Empire, once we were great artists, but now,' Luigo spread his hands and shrugged, 'all we have left is our lifestyle, *bella*. But is a lot! Is the best in the world! And why? Because of *la dolce vita*, which you are living – tasting every day the sweetness of life. This is not about parties or paparazzi ... although,' he winked, 'it is a bit about Marcello Mastroianni ...' We both sighed dreamily, leaning on the bar.

'Is it about Sex du Soleil?' I asked.

'Yes, but not just. It's about tasting the tomato, tasting the kiss, tasting the Venus, tasting the olive oil ...'

'Singing in Pegna?'

'Yes! Singing in Pegna, singing in the rain, singing ... Madonna!' As his idol came on the stereo, Luigo segued expertly into 'Holiiiddaaaaaaay ...' jabbing his fingers in the air to the rhythm.

'Celebraaaaaate!' I jabbed my fingers back at him, wiggling to the beat.

Luigo skipped over from behind the counter in a kicky eighties move and we danced around the bar, serenading each other, and collapsed laughing when the song ended.

Luigo turned to me: 'You see, *bella*? *La vita e dolce* ...'

'Yes, Luigo, yes it is.'

Pasta con pomodoro

Serves 1 (can easily be doubled or tripled or quadrupled)

1 clove garlic
Best-quality extra-virgin olive oil
1 400g tin chopped Italian plum tomatoes
Sea salt
1 large handful spaghetti or other pasta of your choice
Basil, to serve
Parmesan, to serve

Peel the garlic and smash it, using the base of your hand to press down on the flat of a large kitchen knife. Pour a glug of olive oil into a pan and drop the smashed garlic into it. Cook a little – don't let the garlic burn – and open the tin of tomatoes and pour it in. Let it simmer, stirring as it reduces. With tinned tomatoes you only need to cook for about ten minutes.

Fill a large pasta pan with water and put on the hob. Once it is boiling, add some salt and pasta of your choice (spaghetti is a classic, fusilli and penne are also favourites). Stir the pasta when first in the boiling water to stop it sticking together. When the pasta is al dente (usually ten minutes, but taste to make sure it is not overcooked), drain, saving a spoonful or two of water to add to the sauce. Tear up some leaves of basil and throw into the sauce. Take out the clove of garlic and discard. Then add the pasta to the pan of tomato sauce and mix it until the pasta is well covered with sauce, adding a bit of the pasta water if you need to thin the sauce. Grate on a little Parmesan if you wish, then serve.

(Any extra sauce can be kept in the fridge for another day.)

Fennel and blood orange salad

Serves 1, with leftovers

1 big fat bulb fennel, cleaned
2 blood oranges
Best-quality extra-virgin olive oil
Best-quality balsamic vinegar

Chop off the top and bottom of the fennel bulb so you are left with the body of the fennel. Stand it on its bottom and slice in half. Then cut each half into slices – a centimetre or two across – and throw into a bowl. Peel and slice the oranges – I find it easier to slice the whole fruit into 6–8 segments, then cut away the peel. Mix the orange slices with the fennel, add plenty of olive oil, and drizzle on a bit of balsamic vinegar – not too much. Mix it all together and serve.

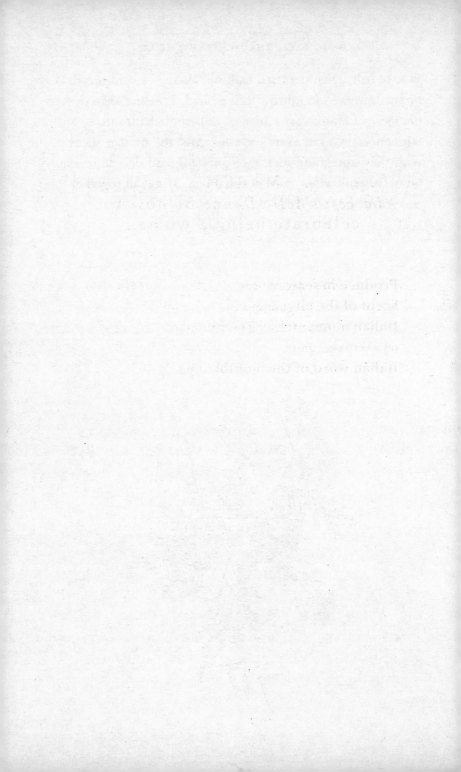

3

MARCH

La Festa delle Donne or how to
celebrate being a woman

Produce in season: peas
Scent of the city: mimosa
Italian moment: riding over the Arno
on a Vespa at sunset
Italian word of the month: *Giaggiolo*

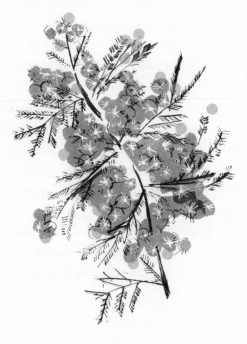

The phone was ringing in the flat as I walked in from the market. I answered, expecting it to be Italian tele-marketeers on whom I had been practising my pigeon Italian. '*Pronto*?' I said.

'Have you fallen in love with Giuseppe yet?' chirped a playful, staccato voice on the other end. I laughed. Christobel, in her official role as my fairy godmother, rang once a week to check up on me.

'No but I think we may be becoming friends,' I said, 'which might be even better.'

Christobel admitted that Giuseppe, with his strange habits and intense privacy, was probably not ideal lover material but would make a loyal friend.

'I was thinking,' Christobel trilled, 'why don't you stay?' In her inimitable way, she had intuited my desire to remain in Florence. I could imagine Christobel sitting at her dressing table, in a black Miu Miu shift and Prada sti-lettoes, her old-fashioned receiver held near her ear so as not to disturb her stripy coiffure. 'I will be coming out now and then but otherwise you can be there. So we were wondering whether you want to? I mean, if you haven't got anything else planned?'

The way I had been living in London now made no sense at all. Work hard during the week and at week-ends have your real life, shopping in a soulless supermar-ket where fruit and vegetables lay on little paper coffins wrapped in plastic shrouds. Now the idea that my work and personal life should be separate was anathema. Office life made no sense any more; even as I had been gripped in its hold, in the affirmation of money and status, the idea that I was spending so many hours every day, the majority of my life, in neon light sitting on my bottom – gathering new fat cells – had been growing distasteful, but I was too busy to think of alternatives and my imagination had been slaughtered by the daily grind. Now that I was living without all the relics of my former identity, there was a glimmer of something new. The heady possibility of freedom.

My only ambition now was to live as well as the Italians.

To my frustration, Beppe was proving hard to pin down. He'd flirt with me at the café but when we'd set up an assignation at my flat he'd fail to turn up. At best he'd text an excuse and at worst not even do that. After the grand high of feeling desirable, it was especially deflating.

'He's scared of you!' pronounced Luigo. He had listened patiently to my nightly reports on the non-progress of our affair, and this was his favourite explanation for Beppe's ambivalence – alongside 'could he be gay?' (Luigo was apt to ask this about any handsome man that came into the bar, the presence of girlfriends notwithstanding). 'He knows you are leaving and he is scared to get involved.'

'But it can't be that, Luigo. I'm only going back to London for two weeks and then I will be back,' I whined. 'Oh God, I forgot to put on a robe when I went to make us some tea. Maybe he saw the size of my bottom and now he will never touch me again …'

Luigo sighed, exasperated: 'Oh *bella*, have I taught you nothing about being a woman?'

One Thursday morning early in March I stumbled upon a flower market in the loggia of the Piazza della Repubblica, the nineteenth-century square built on the site of the city's Roman forum and its old ghetto. Lined by glamorous cafés with large terraces, there was a brightly painted carousel in the middle and a long loggia down one side, a large victory arch connecting the piazza with some of Florence's most expensive shopping streets.

My destination was the city's main post office, and I was anticipating a long morning – this was not my first experience of how hours are lost in an Italian post office, a sort of Bermuda Triangle in which both time and the will to live vanish regardless of the simplicity of the tasks you have to perform. But I forgot about my errand as soon as I stepped in through the columns: there were flowers, blooms and blossoms everywhere. In my single-minded pursuit of more sex with Beppe, I had failed to notice spring's approach but here the new season positively assaulted me. Fragrance burst around me – heady hyacinths, small narcissi full of sweet perfume, and everywhere, thin branches bearing fluffy clusters of yellow mimosa, each one a tiny bomb of delicate scent. Every stall had mimosa covering it, tall branches bowing over the tables or fat bouquets wrapped in yellow ribbon laid out in a row. I paused to take a deep breath, and, quick as a flash, the stallholder put a slim bouquet in my hand. I buried my face in the downy petals, smiling at him broadly as he said: 'For you. A gift! Happy Women's Day.'

That's how I discovered that in Italy on 8 March, women were celebrated with offerings of mimosa. As I walked through the centre back to San Niccolò, I was stopped on the bridge by Old Roberto who pushed on me several small branches of mimosa plucked from his own tree. Giuseppe the Gnarled Jeweller appeared at his door to present me with a small bunch, Cristy put a garland in my hair. The Rifrullo Pavarotti greeted me with a posy and a snatch of song, and Guido the Dramatic Idraulico pressed on me a corsage so pretty I gave him a kiss on the cheek, leaving some gold sparkles on his beaming face. In the *forno* the baker himself appeared and slipped a spray of mimosa into the paper bag containing my loaf and even Giuseppe met me outside our shared front door with a lone stalk of little yellow balls. I was so laden down by the fuzzy yellow flowers that he had to open the door for me. I walked upstairs, wrapped in my own cloud of mimosa scent.

Later the same afternoon, Beppe showed up unexpectedly. '*Auguri, bella,*' his voice crackled over the intercom. '*Ti ho portato la mimosa …*'

I let him in and he walked into the fragrance-filled flat carrying the biggest bunch of mimosa yet. As I placed them in a vase next to the corner sofa, I wondered how many of my celebratory flowers would survive our antics.

Hours later, having been left in no doubt as to the desirability of my soft squelchy body, and somehow with not a single vase of mimosa knocked over, I mounted Beppe's

Vespa behind him, circling my arms around his leather-clad waist. He had persuaded me to accompany him to work, 'to stand where I can look at you'. I agreed – I couldn't resist the prospect of a ride through Florence on a Vespa, and of existing for an evening solely to be gazed at.

We puttered through San Niccolò and past my friends: the Dramatic Idraulico paused in his conversation outside Rifrullo with Pavarotti to wave, Pavarotti bellowing out a snatch of Verdi's 'Libiamo'; Cristy bobbed up and down outside her shop, wearing a spray of mimosa in her hair, her arms open wide as she called out '*auguri!*' Jack the dog barked at us from inside the jewellery shop and as we rounded the corner into the Piazza Demidoff, Old Roberto gazed suspiciously at Beppe as I waved. I felt like the Queen passing through her subjects.

In the middle of the Ponte alle Grazie, Beppe pulled over to one side and turned to me, his helmet framing his handsome face.

'Look, *bella*, especially for you. Happy Women's Day!' He kissed me, pointing to the Ponte Vecchio just downriver, thrown into shadow as the sun set behind it. The cloud-streaked sky ignited above us, oranges and reds turning to mauve, purple and rose, the river flowing like liquid amethyst below. Beppe kicked the *motorino* back to life, his strong back pressing against my belly as I sniffed contentedly at the mimosa pinned on my coat, the sky on fire.

The next Sunday evening, when Beppe failed to ring as promised, I rang Luigo. 'We're going out to have some fun, *bella*. Meet me by Dante in twenty minutes.'

I found Luigo standing by the dour poet and followed him down a side street where he stopped at two tables outside an unpromising-looking bar called, appropriately, Piccolo.

'Here? Really?' I raised an eyebrow.

'Yes really,' Luigo pouted. 'It's quiet now, but it's only nine o'clock.'

He brought us two tall beers outside and thimblefuls of vodka – 'Tonight you drink!' he ordered. It was cold but Luigo had to smoke and so we let the vodka heat us up.

Soon we were joined by Luigo's friends. At the centre of the group was a tall skinny creature of indeterminate age with alabaster skin and scarlet lipstick, ink-black hair falling straight down the shoulders of her fuchsia taffeta ball gown, which was lobbed off at the knee. She was flanked by two beautiful boys at least twenty years younger than her – Luigo whispered that Antonella – Anto – was always accompanied by at least two young Adonises, gay icon of Florence that she was. The puffy sleeves of her dress were so exaggerated they would have been comical on anyone else but she had such an insouciance that she looked, instead, perfectly, ironically, gorgeous.

When she made a throwaway comment – in excellent English – about the inspiration for her outfit being Alexis Carrington Colby, I knew that Antonella and I would be friends. Luigo had been quite right about Piccolo: by midnight the narrow alley was filled by bare dancing torsos and thumping music.

The next day the phone jangled through my hangover. I was lying inert on the sofa making my way through a

pot of tea, wishing it was attached to me by intravenous
drip – the very act of lifting the pot made my head hurt.
The blended perfume of mimosa, hyacinth and narcissus
on my kitchen table was making me feel nauseous.

'*Pronto?*' I whispered.

'*Tesoro*,' the unmistakable husky tones of Antonella
echoed through the receiver. 'Carrington Colby here.
Probably your head hurts.' I nodded. She went on as if she
could see me. 'I think you should come here and have a
coffee. Then stay for lunch. *La mamma* is cooking her hangover cure ...'

I forced myself to bathe and dress. The sun was shining
and I scrabbled to find some sunglasses before I went blind
walking over the river. Antonella lived with her elderly
widowed mother in the piazza of Santa Croce itself, above
a leather shop. I had cut through the alleyway we had spent
our evening in, passing the closed Piccolo with a shudder.

Antonella, who had just turned fifty, was not a standard
Florentine woman of her generation, with their penchant
for navy quilted jackets and classic clothes. She worked in
fashion and her own tastes ran to vintage designer pieces
– she would have been at home in the wilder reaches of
hipster Hackney or Brooklyn's Bushwick. And she had
unfailing style. She oozed it through her hangover today
in black polo neck and ski pants, a huge pair of black sunglasses obscuring half her face, and perfect red lipstick,
looking like Emma Peel from *The Avengers*.

'*Permesso*,' I said as I crossed the threshold, and I could
see from Antonella's smile that minding my manners
was the right thing to do. I had noted the formalities in

Italian culture from my very first trip with Kicca when she greeted people she was meeting for the first time with '*salve*' and not '*ciao*'. She had told me about the correct forms of address, the difference between the formal '*lei*' and '*tu*', how the old-fashioned way – still employed in the south – was to use the very formal '*voi*'. I understood all this instinctively from Iranian culture – I had always used the formal plural to address my parents out of respect.

On entering, I understood why she was wearing her sunglasses indoors – the flat was blindingly bright. It hurt my head. 'Come in, *tesoro*,' said Anto. 'Put those back on,' she pointed to my sunglasses. 'At least till after we have had coffee.' She busied herself in the kitchen, explaining that her mother was at the market, shopping for lunch. I watched her move about carefully preparing the moka, explaining what she was doing over her shoulder, telling me that the coffee maker must never be overfilled and compacted too much, that the water used should never be hot, it should be placed on a low heat and that, above all, as soon as the machine started to splutter, it must be taken off the heat immediately. While coffee was a sacred ritual, Antonella was quick to tell me she could not and would not cook. 'Luckily, *la mamma* takes care of that, otherwise I would be dead!'

She served coffee on a little silver tray, picking out two small wafer-thin china coffee cups and matching saucers, fetching a small silver sugar bowl with matching tiny prongs, and placing on each saucer a silver teaspoon that matched the sugar bowl. She poured hot black coffee into each cup, and carried the tray to the dining table.

That's when I learnt that no matter how bohemian an Italian woman may be, there were rules she would never break. She would never serve you coffee in a big mug plonked unceremoniously on the kitchen table.

The front door clicked as I was finishing my second cup – *la mamma* had arrived. A small stocky woman – typically Tuscan – she walked in already talking. She was wearing a thick grey coat in wool bouclé, a matching hat covering her short hair. I jumped up, whipping off my sunglasses, and shook her hand as Antonella introduced us. *La mamma* kissed me on each cheek, held me to her ample bosom, and then shed her coat and hat, hanging them up in a closet by the front door, teasing her hair in front of the mirror in the hall. With her olive skin and light brown hair, dark blue slacks and sensible shoes, which she swapped for slippers with a high wedge heel, she looked nothing like her geisha-like daughter. She was homely but the brooch on her cashmere jumper and matching gold earrings were a testament to the care she took over her appearance, even as she went into the kitchen and donned an apron, shooing us out of her way.

Antonella took me to her bedroom, which looked out over the Piazza Santa Croce. It was minimal and edgy like Antonella, with white walls and a few pieces of very good black furniture. There was a bed tucked into the corner, a desk at the other end, and a Le Corbusier black leather sofa and cube armchair against the wall. Framed in the two large casement windows was the marble facade of the basilica of Santa Croce, the fine decorative detail around the front door like ribbons of handmade lace, a mass of people milling around on its wide skirt of steps.

'Ah yes, the church,' said Antonella lightly. 'Any pictures on the walls would be an insult to the Temple of Italian Glories.'

Anto had moved in with her mother after her father had passed away five years ago – 'because no one likes to be alone, *tesoro*. Not that she needs me ...' She went on to recount how, in spite of her seventy-plus years and problems with her knees, *la mamma*'s love for life kept her busy: visiting the market every morning, cooking for them both every day and going dancing every Sunday afternoon. 'I think she has a boyfriend,' whispered Antonella, joining me at the window. 'She won't tell me! But I have my suspicions. Look down there!'

She pointed to a small man sitting on one of the stone benches that lined the square below. He was wearing a checked shirt and flat cap, his hands folded in his lap.

'Look, he's always down there when she's just come home or about to leave to go somewhere,' hissed Antonella. 'I think he walks her home and then rests to catch his breath ...'

'Have you asked her?' I peered out of the window, delighted by *la mamma*'s mystery man.

'Yes, but she refuses to tell me!' Anto started laughing and I joined in. I hoped there would be men clamouring to walk me home when I am in my seventies.

Antonella and I laid the table for lunch, and *la mamma* brought out a single iris in a tall slim glass jar. It was a pale powdery lilac with large petals folded down like tongues. She said, translated by her daughter, that she had spotted the first of the Florentine irises flowering by the side of the basilica. '*Giaggiolo*,' she enunciated the Tuscan name, explaining how the fleur-de-lys symbol of the city etched on all the municipal marques – even on traffic barriers and manhole covers – was in fact a *giaggiolo*. 'They grow wild around here, the scent is lovely,' she offered it to me to sniff. 'In April and May the city is covered …'

Our first course was a dense, hearty soup. I watched Antonella pour oil on top of hers and copied her, mixing it in. It was made with chunks of rough-cut vegetables, green leaves, cannellini beans and a texture I couldn't place.

'Bread!' cried out *la mamma* triumphantly. Antonella told me she had bet her I wouldn't be able to guess. 'This is ribollita, a typical Tuscan dish.

'You see, *cara*,' Antonella elaborated. 'You know Tuscan cuisine is what we call *la cucina povera*? It's kind of peasant cuisine, about using all the produce you have, not wasting anything. It is very earthy, not fancy at all …'

La mamma cut in with an indignant shrug as Antonella translated quickly. 'When the produce is as good as ours, there is no need to cover the taste with sauces and cream and butter. Like the French …' she sniffed her disapproval.

La mamma explained to me that ribollita was made over-night for the flavours to settle. 'The longer you leave it the more delicious it is!' It was one of several Tuscan dishes devised to use the local bread that turned rock hard after a day or two as I knew from even the small loaf that the baker put aside for me

'No preservatives, *cara*,' said Anto. 'Like us Tuscan women, you see. No Botox, not like the Romans! Just nat-ural goodness!' She and *la mamma* laughed lustily.

Each bite of ribollita restored me, it was practically like medicine. I took *la mamma*'s warning not to eat too much as we still had a pasta dish coming up.

'While the pasta cooks, we should try these.' *La mamma* placed a basket of perfect pink radishes on the table, the first radishes of the season, she said, and a superior crop. We ate them with no embellishment and in reverential silence – just the sounds of us crunching. They were so peppery, my eyes almost watered. *La mamma* was right, these did deserve to be a course all of their own.

La mamma brought out the pasta dish. Long strands of spaghetti bejewelled by a scattering of bright green peas, Parmesan melting in, accompanied by a green salad and a side of chickpeas. Another reverential hush fell over the table. After second helpings when we had finished it all off, *la mamma* looked at me with a twinkle. 'Are you married?'

'No, *mamma*!' Anto answered for me. 'La Kamin is single like me …' She pronounced Kamin as Hhamin, in the Florentine way that aspirates hard 'c's into 'h's. I puffed with pride at being transposed into Florentine.

'*Allora, non vi preoccupate,*' said *la mamma*, and launched into a story of a friend who had recently celebrated her eightieth birthday. Her dance partner, a widower, had called round in the morning and offered himself as a gift – 'a day of love before we are too old to remember' – and she had accepted. 'It was the best sex she ever had,' said *la mamma* matter-of-factly. 'So don't worry, everything has its season. Even if you are as old as me!' She laughed with gusto, nudging Antonella, who gave her a long look.

Antonella said wryly, 'At least, *cara*, we have something to look forward to.'

I walked home reflecting on *la mamma*'s words. There was no reason to fret over Beppe. More sex was always round the corner – and it could be the best sex of your life. As I traced my way home through back streets grown familiar, I saw wisteria tumbling over balconies and walls, and, cutting through the green patch of the Piazza Demidoff, I passed a profusion of lilac bushes that had suddenly sprung up out of a corner, their sweet smell dispersing the usual stink of dog pee. The four-petalled flowers were so pretty I plucked a few and carried them home, clamped to my nose. As I left the green I saw a long stem of pale lavender *giaggiolo* straight as a sword, surrounded by blade-like leaves. Spring was coming. I was sure *la mamma* was right, everything had its season.

Ribollita

Serves 4–6

350g dried cannellini beans (if using canned beans, use 400g tin of beans, and keep the water)
Best-quality extra-virgin olive oil
1 clove garlic, smashed with a knife blade
1 stem fresh rosemary
Sea salt and black pepper, to taste
2 onions, finely chopped

3 stalks celery
2 carrots
1 potato, peeled and finely chopped
1 savoy cabbage
1 400g tin chopped Italian tomatoes
4 handfuls bietola (Italian chard – you can also
use spring greens)
4 handfuls cavolo nero (Italian kale)
Stale sourdough bread (half a loaf)
Dried red chilli flakes, to taste
Dried thyme, to taste

This soup takes a little preparation but is worth the effort.

Soak the dried cannellini beans in a large bowl of water, preferably for 24 hours but at least overnight. Once the beans have soaked, heat a good glug of olive oil in a large deep pan, then add the clove of garlic and stick of fresh rosemary. Cook for a minute or so (do not let the garlic burn), then add the beans. Then add 2 litres of water – a lot of water is needed. Bring to the boil and then cover and let simmer on a medium-hot heat for an hour. Once the beans are cooked, season with salt and pepper – not before. If using tinned beans you don't have to cook for so long or in so much water.

Remove the stick of rosemary and half the beans and reserve to one side. Keep the rest of the beans in their water – this will be the stock for your soup – and blend

smooth with a handheld blender. If using tinned beans, add
the bean water here.

In a separate deep pan, add a glug of olive oil, then add
the onions, celery and carrots, and sauté until golden to
make a soffritto. Add the potato to the soffritto, stirring
as they all cook. Take the tin of tomatoes and mash them
into a pulp with a fork, then add to the soffritto and potato
cubes. As this mixture simmers, remove the body of the
stalk from the savoy cabbage and finely chop the leaves
into julienne – long, thin slices. Remove the stalks from
the bietola leaves, but chop into large pieces. Do the same
with the cavolo nero leaves. Add all the different leaves to
the soffritto, tomato and potato mixture, stirring together
over the heat. Add the bean broth, cover, and bring to the
boil. Once it is boiling, remove the cover and simmer for
another 45 minutes, stirring frequently.

Fill the bottom of a large casserole/Dutch oven with
chunks of the sourdough bread. Pour half the soup over
the bread. Add another layer of bread and then pour on the
rest of the soup. Let it cool until it is tepid, then cover with
cling film and leave in the fridge for at least two hours. If
you can leave it overnight, don't use the cling film. When
you take it out, the bread will have absorbed the soup.
Return to the pan and heat, bringing to the boil, then season with salt, black pepper, some dried red chilli flakes and
thyme leaves. Serve, pouring on a slick of olive oil once it
is in the bowl.

Spaghetti with peas alla Fiorentina

Serves 4

1 large white onion
Best-quality extra-virgin olive oil
2 cloves garlic
1 kg peas (in shells)
A small handful parsley
Sea salt and black pepper, to taste
Pancetta (50g cut into fine pieces)
Spaghetti (75–100g per person)

Finely slice the onion. Heat a good glug of olive oil in a pan, add the onion, one smashed clove of garlic and cook till transparent. Shell the peas and put them in the pan with the onion. Add another peeled and smashed clove of garlic, and some sprigs of parsley; season with sea salt and a little black pepper. Let it simmer, but before the peas are completely cooked and the water all gone (roughly 10–15 minutes but keep an eye on it), add the pancetta.

At the same time, heat a large pasta pan filled with water and add a generous pinch of salt when the water is boiling. Add the spaghetti and once cooked (al dente), drain, saving some of the pasta water to add to the peas. Add the spaghetti and a cup of the pasta water to the peas and mix it all together till the pasta is covered with the sauce. Serve.

4

APRIL
Fare l'amore or how to take a lover

Produce in season: artichokes
Scent of the city: orange and lemon blossom
Italian moment: kissing in Siena's campo
Italian word of the month: *baciami*

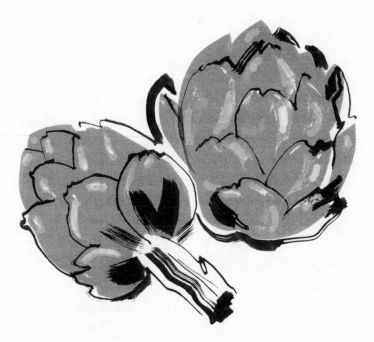

I had just walked into an exhibition in a scruffy part of Santa Croce and was making my way round the artworks, when my phone pinged:

what are u doing 2nite?

It was from Rag-Trade Roberto who I had met the day before; we had shared a table at Cibreo. He had started chatting to me while I worked my way through some mini pizzas that Beppe had pressed on me. He told me he worked 'in the rag trade' and I liked his deep voice, his playful manner. Quite unlike Beppe's vacant stare, Rag-Trade Roberto's eyes had been mischievous and warm, lively and curious behind round spectacles. His flicky brown hair was worn a little long and he sported preposterous sideburns, two triangles of hair trimmed deep into his cheek.

He had asked me where I was from and I had retorted, 'Well, not from the nineteenth century like you,' and he had roared with laughter. That's when I had noticed the gap in his front teeth and all thoughts of Sex du Soleil were forgotten. He was devastatingly sexy, a grown-up, handsome man.

I had given him my number while Beppe had been busy serving a customer.

Now I texted back:

female art show with neighbour
is it glamorous?

I looked around. The neon-lit room was like the classroom of an adult education college. The exhibits – paintings,

collages and even a frame containing little knitted figures —
were pinned up on moveable whiteboard walls. On long
tables, there were paper plates with little piles of crisps
and peanuts; someone had, inevitably, brought hummus.
Moving through all this were scruffy, dirty-haired women
in combats and shapeless hand-knitted jumpers. They were
unlike almost all the other Italian women I'd met.

no I texted back.

is there any food?

not really. Giuseppe said maybe pizza later

basta pizza! Send me the address, I am coming to get u

Ten minutes later a shiny black Audi was purring outside
and Roberto was grinning at me from the open window.
He was wearing a pistachio-coloured cashmere jumper
under a cord jacket, his hair was flicked back off his face.
I caught a whiff of cologne as he kissed me on the cheek
and I inhaled deeply. As I lowered myself carefully down
into the low leather seat, he declared dramatically: 'You
must stop eating like a tourist. All that pizza!' I laughed. 'I
am going to give you a proper meal!'

He turned the full force of his gap-toothed smile on
me and charisma flooded the car. My stomach flipped. I
beamed back and nestled in. We raced through the night
until we drew up outside the centre of the city at a small
restaurant filled with the hum of elegant dining. I had
dressed up my casual outfit with enormous earrings as
usual, but I was dramatically underdressed compared
to the other women there in their silks and furs, hair
groomed smooth, heels sky-high. I took in the scene —
my first proper date at a good restaurant in Florence.

I felt scruffy and unsophisticated and even more so when Roberto was stopped at several tables by polished ladies who pawed at him. He seemed to know – and be loved – by everyone. 'Italian women,' he murmured in my ear, 'never knowingly underdressed ...'

I giggled, liking the hand that touched my back, guiding me through the tables.

Taking my seat, I regaled him with descriptions of the art collective: the adult education classroom, the women in their combat trousers, and the installation that featured several small knitted figures.

'Ah, lesbians!' he declared, nodding sagely. 'Good I came for you!'

He offered to order for me, and I gladly accepted – I didn't understand the menu and it felt so considerate. I watched as he chatted to the waiter about the freshest dishes, what was good that day, barely glancing at the menu as he ordered, the whole process a conversation.

'All the women I spoke to tonight,' I said, 'told me I was mad to leave London and move to Florence. I couldn't understand it.'

Roberto leant in. 'Florence is small, *cara*,' he said. I was leaning in too and could hardly concentrate on what he was saying, his hand on his glass was so thrillingly close to mine. 'You may love it now, like all the tourists, but you'll go home in a couple of months. It's always like that.' He tossed his head as if it was a foregone conclusion.

Before I could protest, he told me that he loved London but could never countenance living there. He was a gourmet. 'You see, *cara*, there is no food culture in England.

People don't know how to eat. They cook boring food or go out for overpriced boring food. And the vegetables ...'

'I know,' I cut in, 'they are tasteless, poor us! But Roberto!' I felt bound to defend my home city. 'It's not like that any more. We have wonderful restaurants in London and TV cooking shows are all the rage, everyone's into Slow Food and organic ...'

'Yes yes,' he dismissed me with a wave of the hand. 'That's the point. To eat well in London it has to be a trend – a movement or fashion. Last time I was there my friends took me to a place, how is called, 'Olefoods. All my English friends so excited – look at the tomatoes they said, just like in Italy. And there were a lot of different sorts, is true. But it was seven pounds for two tomatoes ...'

'I know,' I lamented, 'it's nothing like Sant'Ambrogio.'

'Ah, so you see!' he exclaimed. 'In Italy, eating well is not just for rich people. We Italians like pleasure, *cara*, we are not in love with denial like you English ...'

Right on cue, the food arrived. A plate of mature pecorino cheese with honey from the owner's own beehives over which we both umm'd and ahh'd. The small bowl of steaming tagliatelle with wild boar sauce so rich that on tasting it Roberto closed his eyes in rapture, raising a hand and waving it by his head in that wordless Italian gesture understood the world over. He leant in and told me that he was a hunter himself. 'I love to be on the land, *cara*,' he drawled in a low, intimate voice, as if confiding something very important to me. 'I love to hunt, to fish, to be with nature ...'

I licked my lips. The food was exquisite, and the permission to drool over it a nice novelty too. But most of all I was

finding Roberto's close presence almost overwhelming –
his wit, his lightness, his passion for his food, the way he
had of leaning in and catching me in the beam of his attention, his devastating smile. By the time the main course
came round, I was having trouble breaking eye contact for
long enough to check what I was putting in my mouth.

After our *primi* – which was all the pasta had been – the
largest T-bone steak I had ever seen arrived on a wooden
board, practically bleeding. Small plates of vegetables
accompanied the steak, which Dino – as Roberto now
insisted I call him – carved for us, putting two thick slices
on my plate.

'*Bistecca Fiorentina!*' he announced. 'The traditional dish
of Florence. I think you have been so busy with pizza,' he
twinkled, 'you haven't tried this yet?' He drizzled some
oil on top, piled garlicky spinach and courgettes from the
side dishes on my plate, and urged me to eat. The meat was
thick and tender, the juices swishing around my mouth,
my recent vegetarianism abandoned without a thought.

'The secret to Tuscan food, *cara*,' said Dino, 'is that is all
from here. This meat comes from the Chianina cow – have
you seen them all over the countryside? They are white ...'

I confessed I had yet to leave Florence.

'*Dai!*' he exclaimed. 'Well this cannot be. I am going to
the country this weekend, to a friend's house near a hot
spring. You know there are many in Tuscany? No? Ah yes,
we are very volcanic here you know, *cara*, full of heat ...'
With a wink, he continued enthusiastically, 'It's marvel-
looooous, you must come.'

I demurred. According to Luigo's rules – which he had recently drilled me in, taking pity on my pathetic way with men – I was already being too easy having dinner just a couple of days after we met. I was the prize, I reminded myself, I must not get carried away. With as much conviction as I could muster, I politely declined his invitation.

Italian men don't take rejection personally, Kicca had once told me, and I was relieved to find it so when Roberto skated smoothly over it. He regaled me with tales of his wild past – mentioning more than once that he had been quite the playboy – of his 'tragic' health, the digestive problems that had started when he had been working in America and had finally resolved when he had returned to his beloved Tuscany and the Italian diet. When, over coffee, the talk inevitably turned to love, I told him that I had been single for years, skipping over the Nader episode, which I had resolved to relegate to a parenthesis too. He sighed: 'Ah, we are the same. I have been single for a while also.'

'We are?'

'*Si, cara*, we are both adults and we like to play,' he peered at me over the top of his wine glass. I opened my mouth to protest but he went on. 'Love that lasts for ever I don't know about,' he was now looking me intently in the eyes, 'but I believe in *passion* and in living your passion, whether it lasts ten minutes or twenty years.' I gulped, and he smiled a wicked smile. 'Life is for fun … We both know that it's all a game …'

When I rang Dino the next day from Luigo's bar to thank him for a wonderful dinner, he retorted with a smile in his voice: 'Yes, but did you enjoy *me*?'

He was preposterous and I adored it.

Luigo took one look at my dreamy face when I hung up and put a plate of cold pasta salad in front of me.

'Eat this and come back to earth, *bella*,' he said. 'That was Dino on the phone?'

I nodded.

'So you kissed him?' he quizzed.

'No!' He had ended the evening at my door with a solemn kiss on the forehead and I had floated up to bed on air.

'No kiss and you are like this!' he declared. 'This could be trouble ...'

A couple of days later, on a rainy Thursday afternoon, I got a text.

do you miss me?

I typed back: more than you can imagine ...

DINO: i know

ME: and how much do u miss me??

DINO: probably more than you

ME: PROBABLY??!!

DINO: amore mioooooo: probably cos I don't know if u miss me really ... but is a lovely game. I send you kisses

I was still trying to work out a witty response when another message arrived.

DINO: tomorrow lunch or dinner? don't answer both ... too much

I could see the flared nostrils and the toss of the head. I laughed again. But I must make him wait, I had promised myself – and Luigo – and I had lost so much time to daydreaming of Dino at my desk that I had planned a quiet weekend with my book. I must stay true to my mission.

ME: yes it's a lovely game! Can't do lunch OR dinner but ask me again soon?!

I fervently hoped he would.

The weekend slipped by quietly and there was no word from Dino. I went to the market, flirted with Beppe, walked for hours, and worked at my book but everything felt boring. We are playing a game, I reminded myself – but had I overplayed my hand? So when, on Monday afternoon, just as I was fidgeting at my desk I received a text from him, I nearly punched the air. He blinked first, I was winning!

i have booked my favourite fish restaurant Wednesday night. Don't say no, i won't ask again

I replied immediately:

in that case, yes

The restaurant was outside the city walls, in a neighbourhood of artisans and old silk factories called San Frediano. There was another city gate here through which we walked, his arm draped around me as if we were already lovers. The whole evening was seamless, a gratification of a week of waiting, of putting him off, of saying no. I was prepared for the date this time, wearing a red dress Antonella had chosen for me from her own collection of vintage designers – a genuine Fontana Sisters number – and I felt like a million dollars in it. When I shed my coat inside the restaurant, Dino stepped back, his eyes bright, smacking his lips in appreciation, declaring: '*Bellissima!*'

Sitting at the white-clothed table, he ordered several courses of raw seafood followed by oven-baked mains of the fresh catch of the day of river fish, transported from the owner's own streams on his land. Dino dressed my salad when it arrived, poured me wine and placed tender pieces of flesh smelling of the sea in my mouth, a tsunami of attention. Everything I said he found hilarious, everything I did was charming, all his stories led somehow back to me. I felt like the most beautiful woman in the world.

'Better than pizza, no?' he asked at the end of the meal, and I agreed. I recounted the story of a recent date when I'd been taken for pizza (again, in following Luigo's rules, I had been dating men other than Beppe) by a boy called Giacomo who wanted to split the bill.

'*Amore*, that's what you get for going out with boys,' he said in mock horror. 'From now on you must go out only with me!'

As we walked slowly back to the car, he drew me in close and I leant into the cashmere softness of him. We walked in step and I held my breath, waiting for the kiss that would surely follow. Instead he told me about one of his clients, a cashmere company from Scotland.

'I looove cashmere, *amore*,' he explained. 'I wear nothing else. Even in bed. Don't you?'

'Er, no!' I laughed. 'I don't think I know anyone who does. I am obviously moving in the wrong circles.'

'*Amore*, we must fix this immediately!' he exclaimed. 'Why not come with me tomorrow? I am visiting one of my wholesalers and you can choose anything you want. My gift ...'

My eyes lit up.

'I can't think of anything I'd like more,' I said honestly.

The day dawned sunny and it was nearly warm. I was so excited I could hardly breathe. Dino and I had had two dates and he hadn't kissed me yet, dropping me off last night with a heart-stopping smile and another kiss on the forehead. I had paced the flat in frustration – the actual physical discomfort of thwarted desire – before forcing myself to go to bed. It was the first time I was going to see him in daylight and bags under my eyes would not do.

Now I was installed in his fancy sports car and he was taking me shopping – not for diamonds, admittedly, but for cashmere, which was probably more useful in the changeable April days. Days that were timidly warm alternated with a cold that harked back to midwinter. Showers were followed by sunlight, which shone with a golden shimmer. Its rays had embroidered every bush and hedge with small white flowers, their sweet scent weaving in with the fragrance of iris, which wafted all over the city.

When I came down, Dino was leaning against his car, holding up the traffic. I stepped easily into his open arms and, oblivious to the hooting of other drivers, he embraced me before opening the passenger door. In the car, we grinned at each other. His eyes twinkled behind his glasses, his sideburns had been freshly shaped, his cashmere jumper was a soft dove grey, and his cologne tangy. He was so sexy, so quintessentially Italian, I couldn't believe my luck.

Daytime Dino was more brisk, his phone permanently clamped to his ear as he wove at great speed between lanes on the motorway, steering with one hand. He also managed to hold a cigarette with another, and also keep a hand permanently on my knee – quite how he had so many hands doing so many different things I never really understood, but I did notice with some alarm at one point that he was steering us between two trucks with his knees. 'Business, *amore*,' he rolled his eyes as the phone rang again and again. We drove out into the countryside south of the city, a mesh of motorways cut through a dreamscape of Tuscan valleys until, half an hour later, he drew up at a large warehouse on an industrial estate.

I followed him into a hangar full of designer brands. Dino disappeared into an office, leaving me alone with instructions to pick out anything I like. This should have been a dream; in fact, it probably has been, literally, a dream I've had. In my former life I would have run amok here. But now, I looked around, unable to get excited about anything I saw; even Prada dresses lost their allure on being squeezed in unceremoniously with hundreds of others. Try as I might, I was unable to see anything I wanted. I had to admit the bitter truth: here in Italy, the home of fashion, my shopping habit had died an innocuous death.

Contentment is probably consumerism's biggest enemy and I had accidentally found it here in Florence. After so many years of peddling dissatisfaction to women through the pages of the glossy magazines I edited and contributed to, making sure they felt wanting enough in themselves to keep shopping for absurdly priced designer goods to keep the fashion economy booming, I had fallen in with fashion's ultimate nemesis. Because I felt content with my lot, there was no desire left to compete in a race to display the right labels, to be part of a global hierarchy of fashion status. Now, in San Niccolò, I was part of something that was more fulfilling than wearing the latest, coolest brands. I had a community and connection with people in the city that satiated most of my needs. Here in this warehouse, I found myself fingering clothes only to think, but I don't *need* that.

Dino emerged to find me standing empty-handed among the rails, my tummy rumbling. He was determined to give me something and he headed straight to a rack of cashmere jumpers and pulled one out, trying the colour against my face. It was dark lavender, somewhere between the violet of Florence and the pale lilac of its irises. 'This for you,' he pushed it into my hands, ignoring my protests. '*Amore*, I really insist, you must have it.'

I accepted. It was lovely and more so for being from him. Clutching the soft sweater, I followed him out to the car where he turned to me, taking the last drag on another cigarette. 'Now I am all yours, *amore!*' he said with a big smile, jettisoning the butt. 'I take you to lunch.'

Dino decided that we would have lunch in the country. We drove further south through a landscape of cypress trees and olive groves smattered through undulating hills lit by soft golden light. It was the classic picture-postcard view of Tuscany, and it was gorgeous. Half an hour later, we drew up in an unremarkable village, and walked with his arm around my shoulder to what he promised was a 'marvelloooooous' restaurant on the large central piazza. My heart was thumping as we strolled over the piazza, the urge to kiss him so strong I didn't know how much longer I would be able to hold back. The lunch was indeed marvellous but I barely tasted a thing, the butterflies in my stomach were fluttering so hard. Then Dino pronounced the interior of the restaurant too dark and we decided to have our coffee in the sunshine.

He led me out to a café on the square. I started to order a cappuccino but Dino held up a hand in horror. 'You must never drink a cappuccino after eleven in the morning,' he told me off as if I was a small child. 'It's wrong, milk after food, no no ...' he practically wagged a finger. He ordered me a caffè macchiato caldo – a short espresso topped with a little hot milk. 'Is like a mini-cappuccino but not so evil for your belly,' he said, rubbing my tummy as I tried not to wobble on buckling knees. 'I cannot tolerate even a macchiato after eating. Milk after food is just not done.'

I realised now that the look on Kicca's face when I'd ordered cappuccinos after lunch on our trips to Italy had been barely contained horror, and that her not stopping me had been a great act of love.

He threw back his espresso in one gulp. I sipped at my macchiato, watching him in the middle of the square, smoking a cigarette and talking on the phone. His eyes never left mine. I went out to join him.

'We are so near to Siena that it would be a tragedy not to go,' he said. Then he frowned: 'The problem is I have a meeting in Florence in one hour and we don't have time to do both.'

'Oh, don't worry, another time,' I said, trying to hide my disappointment. 'Let's go back!'

'Maybe I can rearrange the meeting ...'

'Really, it's up to you!'

'Well, it depends ...' and he gave me a long look that hit me in the pit of my stomach.

'On what?' I asked, suddenly shy.

He looked at me, his head cocked to one side, a half smile playing around his lips as he took a step deliberately towards me.

'On this ... *Baciami, amore!*'

There in a pool of sunshine in the middle of the square, he wrapped me in his arms and, finally, he kissed me. Birds sang and a breeze fluttered through the trees. I clung to him, melting into this most delicious kiss. It felt like it went on for ever.

When we eventually came up for air, he licked his lips with relish and gazed at me. Then he kissed me again, lightly, as I struggled to catch my breath. 'Now I cancel ...'

Once he had made his phone call, we were elated, like children given the day off school. We ran back to the car. He reached an arm towards me and I shifted myself to land in the crook of his shoulder as he drove, kissing his cheeks, his neck, his lips as he steered. At each red light we kissed for so long the cars behind us hooted to break us apart. The road climbed up approaching Siena's city walls, the glowing countryside falling away behind us in sun-filled valleys, sparkling in the light. His hand rested on my knee and I sighed audibly. He waved his other hand out of the window. 'My country, *amore*.' He presented it to me with pride, a Tuscan man in his landscape.

I am in love, I thought.

Siena seemed made for Dino and me that glowing afternoon. Now that we had finally kissed, we couldn't stop. His lips seemed made for me, his body the perfect fit for mine and his warmth and affection was so familiar and yet so thrilling that I couldn't believe we were not lovers yet. Perched in that delicious place between burning desire and its fulfilment, we had eyes only for each other. Siena's steep medieval streets may have been thronging with admirers but we hardly noticed them. He held me close, dropping kisses on me like butterflies as we walked. I was not prepared for the beauty of Siena's campo, the vast round centre, a space flanked on all sides by tall medieval palaces, pierced in the middle by a tall skinny tower rising out of the monumental edifice of the Palazzo Pubblico. It was gorgeous and dramatically different to Florence's beauty, and I stood and admired as Dino indicated the various buildings, explaining that this large round space was used as the racecourse for the Palio once a year – Siena's famous horse race.

'I will bring you, *amore*!' he promised. 'In the summer ...'

We settled at a table in the square, both putting on sunglasses against the glare. I hung on his every word and he held my hands and kissed each finger in turn. I was dazzled: by him, by the day, by the Campo, and I couldn't keep the smile off my face. An elderly American couple at the next table leant over and asked us to take their picture. Oozing Italian charm, Dino took the camera and snapped them while making them laugh, giving them – as he told me later – at least one story of an encounter with a real Italian – 'not a waiter singing "O Sole Mio"' – that they could return home with. Taking back his camera, the American man suggested taking a picture of us with my phone. 'You should have a picture, you guys look like movie stars!' he said.

That's exactly how I felt sitting next to my handsome Italian man in our dark glasses, his arm slung easily around me, our smiles luminous – I felt as glamorously Italian as he looked. And I felt like a star, like I radiated allure.

The rest of the afternoon was a massive flirtation through Siena's narrow streets overhung by tall palazzos. We necked in every alleyway like teenagers, browsing the shops, taking in the cathedral with its flouncy decorative façade, Dino regularly breaking away to talk on the phone before coming back to me to kiss the inside of my wrist, stroke my hair. By the time we left, the sun was setting and the day was turning cold. I gave an involuntary shiver. Driving out of the city gates, circling our way down the hill, the sun was sinking slowly in the valleys below us, the light gilding the landscape, a perfect reproduction of the scenery in every Renaissance painting I had seen in the Uffizi. Dino stretched his arm out and I moved in close, drinking in the scent of him.

'*Amore*, you are cold!' he declared dramatically.

Amore, I thought, blissfully. I am his *amore*! He had called me *amore* before but now it felt real. Was there a nicer word in the Italian language, I wondered. I assured him that I was OK but now he had taken it into his head that I would catch a chill if he didn't immediately rectify the situation. The Italians, I had noticed, were not only not stoical about the rain, they had a mortal fear of catching chills. I had lost count of the number of times Cristy had pulled my scarf tighter around my neck, that Antonio in the market had pulled the collar up on my coat. Dino was no different.

He swiftly came off the motorway and went down a small road, pulling over to park on the verge of a narrow country road. '*Eccolo!*' he said, helping me out of the car. I had no idea where we were.

Below us a series of small waterfalls fell into a natural pool, steam rising from the white bubbling water into the darkening sky. The rotten-egg smell of sulphuric water engulfed us. A few people were arranged in the rocks over which the water tumbled. 'Come, *amore*, we take a bath. This will cure you of the cold, they are hot mineral waters, they make sure you don't get sick.'

'Dino, but what do we wear?' I cried; we had nothing with us.

'*Boh!*' he threw up his hands. 'Underwear?'

For a moment I paused. 'Perhaps we should come back another time. I mean …' What did I mean? I was not yet ready to take my clothes off in front of him. I felt really shy.

He stopped my words with a kiss. 'Shhh, *amore*, don't stress … we have fun, OK?' He started shedding his clothes and I followed suit, peeling off the layers quickly and following him as he ran through the chilly air and into the warm stinking waters. The water was blissful, cloudy and quite hot, the smell at first almost overwhelming but the feel of it soft against my skin. We paddled around the various pools, finding small waterfalls to lie under, letting the water cascade over our shoulders. He swam around me, coming to lie between my legs where the pool was deep enough for the water to cover us, touching and stroking me all over under the opaque white steaming water, pushing his body against mine, kissing me until I was panting. Meanwhile night fell and the moon rose bright, the steam rising like mist. Soft warm water lapped at our necks, the sounds of the night chirped around us. He was still caressing me under the water, whispering into my ear '*amore, bella ...*' while I gasped.

Eventually he prised his body away from mine. We were quite alone. With a thick voice, Dino suggested we leave – 'if not is too much. *Ma amore, quanto sei bella ...*' We ran out into the cold air, our bodies actually steaming with the heat of the mineral water, so warmed from the waters and our passion that we did not feel the cold, and he handed me a couple of cashmere jumpers he had found in the back of the car, saying: 'We have no towel, use these, they are old samples ...'

I actually pinched myself. Here I was with an Italian playboy in the velvety Tuscan night, being kissed out of my mind and drying myself on cashmere. Drunk with desire, we stumbled back to the car, where he wrapped my wet head in his orange hunting shawl, pulling it tight around my shoulders: 'you must not catch cold,' he said, kissing me all the while. Lying back in my seat, I watched the lights of Siena pass on the hill, the country around us dark and alive, my brain a mush of contentment.

As we drove, the moon illuminated a hilltop settlement that rose up like a mirage. 'Monteriggioni!' Dino pointed – a medieval fortified village, circled by perfectly preserved walls punctuated by watchtowers, lit up like a theatre set. I expected Rapunzel to appear at the small window in one of the towers. '*Amore*, you must be hungry. Florence is far, let's stop here for dinner.'

I acquiesced. This date, this day, seemed to be going on for ever and I was happy for it to. I wanted to stay in this dream for as long as possible. We entered through the city gates into a medieval piazza edged by splendid stone buildings with terracotta roofs, lit up and deserted. At one end of the square there was a restaurant and at the other a hotel. We looked at each other and the question hung unspoken between us. He tucked my hand in his arm and led me to the restaurant. As we ate a typical Tuscan dinner of wild boar pasta and *bistecca*, he consumed me with his eyes, his look reminding me of our passion in the pools of Petriolo, the feel of his skin, silky and stretched over hard muscle, and I longed to touch him again.

Reading my thoughts, he said, 'You know it's getting late ... there is a hotel there ... maybe we should stay.' He was forcing a casual tone into his voice. 'I am tired and is a long drive,' he said, watching me carefully.

I busied myself with my food, suddenly self-conscious. In the moment he had said what I too had been thinking,

I suddenly craved the comfort of my flat, sitting warm in the corner of the sofa with Giuseppe's shadow on the wall opposite. I looked around the trattoria with its boars' heads and hanging legs of ham and, desire turning to inexplicable panic, I wondered if I was safe in his hands.

He frowned at my silence, his face clouding over. '*Vabbé*,' he shrugged. 'Let's finish our dinner and then you can decide.'

I smiled at him shyly.

'Anyway, you have already decided,' he growled, an edge to his voice. I shifted uncomfortably. 'Women always do. But is OK, you can pretend for now …'

It was the first bum note and anxiety gnawed at me. Surely I should be allowed to apply the brakes if that's what I wanted? Or had I already gone too far? I picked at my food, confused, and he excused himself and went to the loo. Quickly I pulled out my phone and texted Giacomo the Pizza Boy, telling him that I would love to have lunch the next day – he had been asking me out ever since our pizza date. I added casually that I was being a tourist in Monteriggioni and to send a search party if I didn't reappear, adding *LOL*. I stuffed the phone back into my bag. This way, should Dino turn out to be a crazed killer, someone would at least notice my absence the next day and know where to look for me. It was a sensible thing to do. Especially when Dino suddenly felt so dangerous.

When he came back he had regained all his charm and we savoured dinner, washed down with superlative red wine. The wine relaxed me and when we fell back out, giggling, into the piazza, he led me to the hotel. 'Let's see the price, *amore*, if it's reasonable we can stay.' He had made the decision.

The receptionist looked at me narrowly over his glasses – no suitcases, no passports. I wanted the ground to swallow me up. When Dino came and took my hand, I noticed he had also managed to procure two toothbrushes, packaged with tiny tubes of toothpaste. Without a word, he took me up to our room, waiting for the receptionist to leave before pushing me forcefully on to the bed. Any protest stayed in my throat as he manoeuvred his body on to mine, kissing me all over, his fingers mapping my body as somehow my clothes came off. He stood over me then, naked, his torso smooth and muscled, his arms beautiful and strong. '*Bellissima sei*,' he murmured, his elegant tapered fingers cupping my breasts, circling my waist, dipping between my thighs, his body engulfing me. The conflagration was intense – no Sex du Soleil, this was deep and serious, all playfulness gone, his eyes never leaving mine as he moved above me, pinned me down and held my wrists.

I swooned under his kisses all the while struggling against the force he was using, instinctively fighting him back, not sure if we were playing or battling each other, but this made him more insistent, more rough, and he pushed himself into me as I gasped, clawing at him, biting his lips, digging my nails into his back, drawing blood. 'Give in,' he whispered, his eyes boring into mine, '*amore*, give in, you are mine. You cannot win!' and as I lost myself to his rhythm, I gave in. It was only in the early hours, as we lay exhausted, his back raw from my scratches, his lips bruised, that he grew gentle again, holding me to him tenderly, muttering '*amore mio*' into my neck as we lost consciousness, entwined.

'Luigo, it turns out I am easy after all!' I announced as I walked into the bar the next evening.

'I knew there was a reason I loved you so much, *bella*,' he said without missing a beat.

As I described the twenty-four-hour date with Dino, Luigo whistled. 'Well, well,' he marvelled. 'He really is a hunter!'

'What do you mean?' I demanded. I had not mentioned his forcefulness; in fact, I had skimmed over it in my own mind; he had been so tender the rest of the night that I convinced myself I had just misunderstood the strength of his passion, and how it had brought out my own wildness.

'He brought out the big guns, no?' Luigo waved the ubiquitous tea towel around. 'Fashion, Siena, the hot baths, Monteriggioni! No wonder you couldn't resist!'

'Luigo, I am in love!' I twirled around the empty bar. 'I know it's early days but I really am in love!'

'What you are feeling, *bella*,' said Luigo sternly, 'is not love. Trust me, this is not coming from here,' he put his hand on his heart.

'Oh, shut up!' I put my hands over my ears and shook my head, singing loudly: 'lalalalaLA I can't hear you ...'

'*Va bene*,' he hugged me. 'Enjoy, *bella*, it sounds like a lovely story.'

Dino and I were speeding along the Lungarno to 'a little family place you will love'. He had come to the flat straight from work and we had spent so long making love that he was worried we would be too late for dinner. '*Amore*, we must eat something light,' he announced as I poured myself into his car, 'it is late and our stomachs cannot take pasta at this hour.' He rang ahead to order. 'Omelettes with fresh *carciofi* – how you say,' he paused to think of the word. 'You know, the vegetable with a heart.'

I laughed – even vegetables had a heart in Italy! 'Artichokes?'

'*Siiiiii, amore*,' he drawled, reaching over to stroke my cheek. 'You are clever as well as beautiful.'

The trattoria was in a tiny side street behind the loggia of the Uffizi, right by the river, at the foot of the Ponte Vecchio. It was cave-like, reached by steep stairs that descended into a small cellar crowded with tables, the walls lined with bottles of wine. Dino was greeted warmly by the owner who showed us to the end of a long table in the corner lined by benches. The omelettes arrived immediately, fluffy and creamy, filled with fresh artichokes – they were now in season, I was told, as he poured me a small glass of wine, urging me to try it, dressing a salad of tender raw artichoke with Parmesan, tearing up chunks of bread with which to mop up the egg. He sat close to me on the bench, our shoulders touching as we ate. Only after we had finished did he ask pointedly about my day. I told him I had seen Old Roberto on the street, and done a little writing, danced with Luigo in the bar.

'And Pizza Boy?' He was watching me. I had confessed to him in the morning that I had a lunch date with the guy who had tried to split the bill, lied that it was long-standing.

'Oh, well, we had lunch and then I went home. That was it,' I said airily.

'Did you kiss him?' His eyes bore into mine.

'Nooooo!' I cried, but my expression flickered and he gasped dramatically.

'*Amore*, you kissed him! You are a terrible liar!'

'Oh, OK, but really he just kissed me at the door and then I ran away, honestly. That was it.' A flash of something I interpreted as pain shot across his eyes before he adopted an impassive expression. I took his hands. I felt awful.

'Dino, oh dear, no, I am sorry,' I said quietly. 'It isn't like me, I promise. Please forgive me.'

'It's really not my business, *amore*, if you want to play it like that ... But don't forget I play the game very well, maybe better than you ...'

'Oh no, I am not playing, it's not a game. I have hurt you and I hate myself,' and I burst into tears of regret. I was filled with foreboding, a sudden terrible fear of losing him.

He softened, taking me in his arms and wiping away the tears. 'Don't cry, my Kamin. Is nothing. But promise, from now you kiss only me.'

'Oh of course, Dino, I promise.'

It was the day before I was flying back to London. I needed to vacate the flat for two weeks – Christobel and her family were visiting for Easter and I was going home to see everyone and fetch more clothes.

Dino bundled me into his car in the morning. 'I take you shopping, some essentials to take home to your *mamma*!'

We drove to the edge of the Cascine Park, the green lungs of Florence. Ahead of us was the Stazione Leopolda, an old train station which had been converted into a vast exhibition space. A large poster advertised a food and wine fair.

We entered the yawning interior of a hall set with rows of stands covered in linen cloth, filled with people. There were food producers from all over Italy, displaying their wares on stalls groaning under elaborate displays and tasting tables: giant rolls of cheese, hams hanging from hooks, rows of slim salamis and fat mortadella, the whizz of meat cutters and clatter of voices, an assortment of smells. Each region was represented, each wine demarcation had its own area, and Dino led me through it all, announcing that our lesson would start with the most precious of all Italian commodities: olive oil. He urged me first to try several types from different provinces of Italy, tutoring me to recognise the various flavours, the rougher taste of oil from the south, the more refined taste of Tuscany's own. I tried to impress him with the knowledge I had gleaned from Antonio in the market, but he looked at me with pity. 'Not too bad, but you still have much to learn,' he said. We tried different oils, dipping fat chunks of bread into saucers bearing golden liquid, rejecting a peppery oil from Sardinia, a bitter oil from Calabria, and finally agreeing on a bottle of greenish-gold liquid with a velvety texture from a farm in Tuscany. I blanched when I saw the price but Dino did not bat an eyelid, pulling out a pile of cash and refusing to let me carry the bag.

We lingered at artisan chocolates and towers of panettone before stopping at a stall with bottles in varying shades of deep brown. My next lesson was in balsamic vinegar.

'This,' declared Dino, 'is the best balsamic in Italy!' The girl
behind the stall nodded and gave me a talk on her wares
in English. I learnt that balsamic vinegar – which should
always be from Modena – was made from the boiled-down
concentrated sweet juice of white grapes. She pointed to
a small bottle filled with what looked like molasses; it was
premium balsamic, aged for five decades in a sequence of
barrels each made from a different wood. It was not vinegar as I knew it; the texture was thick, treacly, an exquisite
blend of sweet and sour. She showed me how to identify a
good balsamic: swirl it around in the bottle, looking for
a consistency that was not too syrupy and not too thin.
The label, she added, has to say *aceto balsamico tradizionale
di Modena*: 'Without this exact wording, they are ordinary
wine vinegars flavoured with caramel or sugar.' We put
away the fifty-year-old balsamic in its delicate little bottle,
and plumped for something more reasonably priced, aged
five years. Again, Dino pulled out his wad of notes and, taking the bottle, guided me towards the Parmesan section.

Here fortresses of cheese rose up like battlements. The
smell was heavenly, I felt like Alice falling down a rabbit hole
made of rich and ripe Parmesan. Golden circles of cheese
sat on each stall, their sides stamped with the marking
Parmigiano-Reggiano. 'This is the third thing you need.' Dino
helped me to a square of cheese from the samples at the
front of the table. Crumbly and moist, it was creamy on the
tongue, nothing like the dried-out Parmesan I was used to.
'Did you know, *amore*, that it takes five hundred litres of milk
to make one wheel of Parmesan?' asked Dino. Well no, I said,
I didn't. 'That weighs thirty-five kilos,' he said, pointing to

one. 'That flavour comes from all that milk, and also because
it's aged for two years.' The man behind the stall chimed in
with: 'It's very good for you as well – it's a good source of
phosphorus, and also protein and calcium ...'

'For seven hundred years, they produce it like this,'
Dino picked up the thread, not to be outdone. 'They add
nothing, just rennet, and then let age for a year and a half.
It has to be stamped on the side so you know is real demarcation.' I looked at him blankly. '*Amore*, our food traditions
are old and very important to us,' he explained patiently, as
if to a child. 'When you have special things – like Parmesan
that has to be made in certain parts of Parma and Reggio-
Emilia only – they are to be respected. Not just for the
history of this food, but is also respect for yourself, for
the people who make it. To you English this is just to fill
your stomach so you can drink more ...' he regarded me
mischievously. 'But for us Italians, our food is an art and
deserves respect, just like your body and what you put into
it. Is – 'ow you call it – a virtuous circle ...'

He asked for some wedges of the cheese to be cut direct
from the wheel, and they were wrapped in greaseproof
paper, and then in a generous roll of foil – this, I was told,
was how I had to store it too. 'Finally,' he told me with a
flourish as he produced his banknotes again, 'remember is
better on pastas that use butter instead of oil, and never
with seafood ...'

I hugged him. 'This is so generous, Dino, thank you!
Why are you so sweet to me?'

He regarded me tenderly. 'Because, *amore*, I see that you
need sweetness.'

Artichoke omelette

Serves 1–2

1 large fresh artichoke
Best-quality extra-virgin olive oil
2–4 eggs depending on size (free range and
    organic)
Milk (2 cups to each egg)
Sea salt and black pepper, to taste
Parsley, to garnish

Take the artichoke and cut away all the hard tops of the leaves. Slice the remaining heart and tender leaves. Heat the olive oil in a frying pan and toss the artichoke pieces in it until a little browned. Whisk the eggs in a bowl with some full-fat milk. Add to the browned artichoke and cook, seasoning with sea salt and black pepper.

When the eggs begin to peel away from the side of the pan, use a large flat wooden spatula or spoon to flip the omelette. Cook the other side until golden, then serve, sprinkling some fresh chopped parsley on top.

Young artichoke and Parmesan salad

Serves 2

3 large fresh artichokes
Thin slices of very good, aged Parmesan

Best-quality extra-virgin olive oil
Balsamic vinegar, to taste
Sea salt and black pepper, to taste

Take the artichokes and slice off the outer leaves and the hard tops. Finely slice the remaining artichokes on to a serving dish and add the Parmesan. Dress with a generous amount of olive oil and a splash of balsamic vinegar, scrunch some sea salt on top, grind in black pepper, and serve.

5
MAY
Mangia mangia or how to eat and not put on weight

Produce in season: broad beans
Scent of the city: iris and acacia
Italian moment: San Niccolò is my outdoor office!
Italian word of the month: *stringimi forte!*

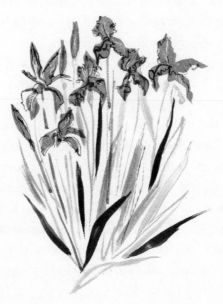

I settled into the seat, fastening my seatbelt. I took out my phone and flipped it open, launching the camera, peering at myself in the small screen. Hair newly trimmed, skin OK for having combatted two weeks of cold in London. I slicked on some of my gold-flecked gloss and pinched my cheeks to heighten the colour – a tip that Luigo had stolen from Scarlett O'Hara and passed on to me – and puckering my lips into a kiss, I snapped a picture. I sent it to Dino.

Seconds later, a reply.

as usual you are most beautiful when kissing me. amore, I come to get u

Two weeks apart and within a couple of hours I would see Dino again. I smiled to myself as I sank back in my seat – I was going back to Florence and my lover was coming to pick me up at the airport. Four months after first arriving there, unaccountably overweight, spotty, burnt out and unhappy, I was going back a stone lighter, a dress size smaller, with not a mark on my skin and joy in my heart. Had I not known it myself, the transformation had been pointed out to me again and again in London; even my mother had looked at my figure approvingly. They asked me what diet I had been on, which new exercise regimen had had this effect, but I was at a loss to answer them – they couldn't believe that a daily dose of pasta, olive oil, red wine and *gelato* could succeed where so many diets and nutritionists had failed. Kicca had shrugged. 'Perhaps it's happiness?' And right now, as I twitched with excitement, this seemed the most likely explanation.

The seatbelt sign lit up; we were ready to land. I looked down at the lights of Pisa – somewhere down there, he was waiting for me. And in Florence, all my friends were doing the same. I had been surprised to receive a text from Beppe while I was away, reiterating his offer to come to the airport to 'carry your bags'. Giuseppe had written regularly with news of San Niccolò. Luigo and I had even sung some Culture Club together over Skype one quiet night.

I was most surprised by Dino, whose ardour had not been cooled by our separation. He had called me every morning as he drove to his 'hoffice' – the family apartment he used for his business – and during the day when he was alone at his desk, he would seek me out on Skype. Our messages often gave way to video calls, and I would shut myself in my room at my parents', enthralled by his face on the screen. It had taken a day or two before our banter had taken a sexual turn, and he had started to demand that I strip off for him. I had complied only when he promised to do the same, and from there it was a small step to the inevitable – video sex. This soon became a regular interlude in our days apart, a compulsion neither of us could resist. I would emerge from my room afterwards, flushed, feeling like the naughtiest girl in school. One day he had regarded me closely across the continent. '*Amore*, your nails are black!' he exclaimed.

None of my previous boyfriends had looked at me so comprehensively, so exhaustively, none had been so vocal on my appearance, so involved with what colours I wore or what I should be eating.

I held out my hands to the camera. 'Do you like it?'

'Hmmm,' he pondered. 'I preferred the one you had on before. You should get some of the Chanel beige, is so elegant, would look marvelloooooous on you, *amore*.'

'Yes, but this colour is very fashionable right now,' I countered.

He held out a hand. '*Amore*, I cannot discuss fashion with an Englishwoman!'

I burst out laughing. His most arrogant declarations always made me laugh the most. I challenged him. 'Oh, come on, give us Brits our due. Look at Vivienne Westwood,' I pointed out. 'No one cuts a suit like her—'

'No, really, *amore mio*, I cannot have this conversation. I am Italian …'

Now, on the plane, I looked at my hands, my nails painted classic Chanel beige. He was right, it was more elegant, but I had packed my black nail varnish anyway.

But first I needed to arrive, to see him, to reconnect with him after our disembodied talks and removed intimacy. My stomach was churning with anticipation. I jiggled impatiently through landing, disembarkation, while waiting for my luggage and passport control. Through to the arrivals hall and there he was, standing right in front of the door, small and compact in jeans, a polo shirt and coral cashmere jumper, his hair flicked off his face. Dino! In all his glory, his chestnut-brown hair a little shorter than before, his absurd sideburns a little fatter, his eyes glittering with welcome. He opened his arms and I fell into them, burying myself in the intoxicating cashmere softness of him, the warmth of his skin, the hardness of his body.

He crushed me into him, kissing my neck, my cheeks, my lips over and over again, holding my face in his hands and drawing back to look at me, examining every feature.

'*Amore*, you are so much more beautiful without pixels,' he exclaimed and my nervousness disappeared. 'Now,' he said, picking up my cases, 'I think first you need a good Italian meal to help you recover from tasteless British tomatoes.'

'*Baciami!*' I leant towards Dino, lifting up my face to his.

We were in Nello, a plain country restaurant in a village twenty minutes south of Florence, where we were now regulars, and Dino had started my Italian lessons.

'First, the first person singular of the verb *avere*?' he said, pointing to a paper placemat which he had filled out with columns of Italian verbs and some phrases he considered essential:

baciami – kiss me

non smettere di baciarmi – don't stop kissing me

abbracciami – hug me

stringimi forte – hold me tight

I couldn't be bothered to conjugate verbs when it was so much more fun to tease him. '*Abbraccia mi*,' I sidled up to him.

'No, conjugate *essere*, I insist!' he tried again.

'*Stringimi forte* …' I leant my head on his shoulder.

He shrugged dramatically and wrote out another phrase on the placemat: *vorrei un po' di pane*.

'I would like some bread,' he said. 'This one is more useful.'

'*Stringimi forte* …' I said again, leaning into him.

'If you are not going to take this seriously,' he pretended to be cross, 'how can you expect to impress the baker?'

'But Dino, what use do I have for bread when I could live on *baci*? If only you would *non smettere di baciarmi.*'

He laughed, giving up on Italian lessons, and kissed me instead over our simple dishes of spaghetti with the courgettes that had just started appearing in the market.

Dino and I were a couple. We had been inseparable since I had promised to kiss no one but him, notwithstanding my time away, and indeed, I had kissed no one but him. He rang as soon as he woke up in the morning and my day was peppered with his texts and calls until we met in the evening. This, I was sure, was love. No one had ever paid such intense attention to me before and if there was even a small crack left in my heart from its shattering by Nader, it had been healed a hundred times over.

One Saturday morning at the beginning of the month soon after I got back, Dino called.

'*Amore*, I am at my tennis club, but I shower and I fly to you,' he said. He was often at his tennis club – his toned arms and abs bore testament to this – and his favourite activity had become flying to me. 'Be ready in half an hour,' he ordered.

He had grown bossy outside of bed too and I adored it. It made me feel feminine, wanted.

Half an hour later, as promised, I found him waiting for me by my door, smoking. Across the road stood Old Roberto, also smoking, and glaring. I waved to him. 'Come on,' I said to Dino, 'there's someone you should meet.' We crossed the road and I introduced him to the old man who looked him up and down with naked animosity.

'Ah,' he said accusingly, turning to me as if he understood at last. 'So, you have a younger Roberto?'

Dino looked at me quizzically, and bidding the old man a good day, we jumped into the car and zoomed away into the hills.

I filled Dino in on how one day while visiting his garden, Old Roberto had proposed marriage to me, and how I had laughed in his face. 'But he was being serious, Dino – can you imagine?' I had picked up this verbal tic from Dino – the constant amazement at things that were unimaginable. In fact, my whole life right now felt like something that until lately was unimaginable, and I truly was in an almost constant state of amazement.

He nodded sagely. 'Yes, I am not surprised.'

'Dino! It's absurd, he's a hundred years old, how could he have been serious?'

'Let me explain to you, *amore*,' he said. 'Of course he was serious; Italian men will always try for a beautiful woman; we appreciate beauty, age has nothing to do with it.'

'But for goodness' sake …' I protested.

'Listen,' he interrupted me. 'I tell you about Italian men. Love and beauty for us is not a joke, is very serious. Maybe the only serious thing. I see you have been kind with that sad old man, you are such a sweet girl. But of course he hopes that he can have you, this is just logical. It's the law of averages.'

'Well, that doesn't make me feel very special,' I laughed.

'No no, you misunderstand,' he cried. 'A woman's beauty for us is always compelling. So we try. With everyone. And like this, someone will say yes!'

I chewed this over. 'Now I feel bad I hurt his feelings.'

'No, *piccolina*, *mai*!' he assured me, squeezing my knee. 'We take rejection very well. We are very used. If she says no, *vabbé*, maybe the next one will say yes!'

'Dino – so if I had rejected you,' I pressed on, 'you would have just shrugged and tried with the next girl you saw?'

'*Nooooo, amore, certo che no!*' he cried dramatically. 'If you had said no, I would have crawled home and died of a broken heart.' He smirked, flaring his nostrils, flicking his hair.

I started laughing. 'Yes, OK, you would have wasted away on a pile of cashmere and your sideburns would have wilted ...'

He was laughing too now. 'Ah, *amore*, you know me so well.'

I needed to know more.

'You know what they say about Italian men,' I asked him, 'that they are all vain mummy's boys who just lie and cheat on their women and care more about how they look than being a responsible partner – is it true?'

Without missing a beat, he replied, '*Ma certo!*'

I was taken aback. 'What, you too?'

He was looking at me with a grin I couldn't read. '*Amore, ma si*, is true of all. Of course I am a terrible liar. I told you before, never trust an Italian man!'

I couldn't tell if he was joking and my heart was suddenly beating very fast. 'Are you lying to me now?'

He laughed uproariously as he pulled over to park. '*Dai, piccolina!*' He took my head in his hands and dropped light kisses all over my face. 'No, I have never lied to you, and I will not lie to you. But I am telling you how it has been ...'

'So you are a reformed character?'

'This you know already. No more playboy. I want a quiet life in a stone house in the country, with dogs and wild boars I can shoot from the window ...' He gave me his gap-toothed grin and I decided to believe him.

I was sitting outside Rifrullo. May was my favourite month so far. The back wall was embroidered with jasmine, its fragrance drifting to where I was bent over my computer. The trees outside the gate were also in flower, acacia hanging like bells from the branches, their aroma combining with the jasmine. I sat out here on fine mornings with a cappuccino and my laptop, working, watching life on the corner, bathing in the sweet soft air.

My street had turned into an open-air theatre – life was now lived outside. Cristy had emerged from behind the counter of her shop and stood at the doorway, bobbing up and down when a familiar face walked by. Even Giuseppe the Gnarled Jeweller was out walking Jack the dog round the block instead of hiding in the depths of his shop by the heater. Old Roberto lingered longer than usual on street corners, parking himself by the jasmine and bending down to drink from the fountain set into the wall. He filled his cupped hands with water that, he told me, once flowed straight from the hills. Old Roberto was more voluble than usual. He, like everyone else, was infected with

this mild spring fever, a feeling of waking from hiberna-
tion, the return of life out of the huddled interiors and
into the open, under the sun, a preview of the summer to
come.

The via di San Niccolò was a stage, and Dino and I had
taken our place in the neighbourhood tableau as The Lovers.
Whether stopping at Rifrullo for a mid-morning coffee or
sitting outside the wine bar just outside the city walls, we
were always together and always intertwined. I was not
used to such public displays of affection. But Dino had no
such compunction, wrapping me in his arms as we sat sipping our coffees, holding my hand as we bought bread in
the *forno*, giving me long kisses as we ordered lunch. All
but the most intimate parts of our love affair were acted
out in San Niccolò. This is how I learnt that in Italy, love is
always a cause for celebration – the more affectionate we
were, the more excitedly we were received, and I felt like
a celebrity when I had Dino by my side. Like the jasmine
on Rifrullo's back wall, I bloomed in the warmth of Dino's
attention, losing my reserve and playing my part in the
tableau almost as enthusiastically as he did.

I was surprised that my body was still shrinking. Every
night Dino took me to a different trattoria out of town,
sometimes in Chianti, sometimes near Florence in the
hills to the south. Plain brightly lit village eateries or cavernous country places hung with hams; either way we ate
beautifully. Many of our evenings were spent in Nello,
where Dino talked for so long to the waitress that sometimes
I thought she was going to draw up a chair and sit down.

Sometimes we were joined by his friends, and Dino spent the first course translating for me until their discussions grew heated and he paused only to say: 'As with all Italians when they get together, *amore*, we are talking about food!' No one seemed to mind him nuzzling me at the table; in fact, they delighted in it, kissing my hand on saying good-bye, patting him on the back with a congratulatory '*Grande Dino!*' I stopped being shy about displaying our relationship so publicly.

Whether we were alone or with friends, the courses arrived one after the other, all on small oval plates; even the pasta dishes were delicately served in small portions, disabusing me of my misconceptions about Italian food, of the idea that eating multiple courses had to be fattening. I used to think of Italian food as consisting just of pasta, pasta and then more pasta. For a change from pasta, there was pizza. All calorie bombs, right?

Wrong.

I discovered with Dino that while Italians did eat pasta and even pizza, these were nothing like their northern European and American counterparts. Pasta servings were small, pizzas had wafer-thin bases, toppings did not include meatballs or chunks of roast chicken, and definitely not pineapple. Typically, an Italian meal consisted of multiple courses. The first – *antipasti* – was hors d'oeuvres, a starter dish smaller than those on our menus. This was followed by the *primi* – the first course, which was pasta, gnocchi or risotto – although risotto not being a Tuscan dish, it hardly ever appeared on the menu. The *secondi* was the meat or fish course and was accompanied by *contorni*, side dishes of vegetables and salad. Lastly there was the *dolci* – dessert – and most meals were rounded off by a short dark coffee – espresso for us but in Italy just *caffè*. We adhered to multiple courses but the curious thing was that at the end of the meal, I was never stuffed, just pleasantly full.

Eating with Dino, flirting and laughing our way through the meals, I ate slowly, each meal drawn out as much for the pleasure of the company as for the pause between the end of one course and the arrival of the next. The brain had time to realise how full it was, so there was no overeating. I had found my natural limit again. Never previously known to willingly turn down a tiramisu, I now often chose fruit or nothing at all. The majority of our meals were made up of salads and vegetables, and Dino explained that having so many different tastes on the table stimulated and satiated the taste buds.

Now my windows were often open, the sounds and the smells emitting from my neighbours' homes made my mouth water – the preparation of food, accompanied by the musical cadence of Italian, the fizz of a fryer, the bubble of boiling water, but most of all, the scent of all those flavours and ingredients coming together. I was inspired to try out the new vegetables I had found in the market, sometimes spending a whole morning shelling broad beans so I could serve them to Dino for lunch with pecorino cheese, as recommended by Antonio.

I nosed round the market every morning, opening my basket for Antonio to fill with the new season's goodies: purple-veined radicchio, peppery, dark wild rocket. I learnt to grill radicchio and sauté cicoria with lemon and garlic. I made a salad of wild rocket with slivers of the exquisite Parmigiano that Dino bought me. I also made the Dramatic Idraulico's tomato sauce regularly, and was now bold enough to start it off with a few diced vegetables – onions, carrots and celery as advised by the market gang, a *soffritto* – the holy triumvirate of Italian cooking, the base of many dishes. Antonio had explained that onions added richness, carrots sweetness and the celery a sort of savoury taste that the Japanese call umami.

Dino never stayed the night although we spent most of our evenings together and he often dropped by during the day – I had grown proficient at Love in the Afternoon. One afternoon, he caught me trying to replace a screw that had fallen out of the wall. He took over and fixed the fallen picture back in place. Then he took my face in his hands and enunciated slowly: '*Amore*, you can ask for help. You are not alone, I am here.'

Not alone. I had been so used to doing everything alone for so long, and after the affair with Nader I hadn't imagined that I would ever dare connect with a man again. Was Dino really here for me? I wondered. 'Come on, *amore*,' he said, leading me out of the flat, 'I want to show you something special.'

He drove up to Piazzale Michelangelo, pulling over in the far corner of the car park and jumping up to open the car door for me. He led me to the stone balustrade, pointing down to a garden that fell away below us, roped-in flowerbeds crowded with tall iris flowers. Bigger than the size of my hand, they displayed the most psychedelic

colour combinations: flame-orange frills with a white
tongue, an inky dark blue, a bridal white with layers of
frills; there was even a black one, its velvety depths dark
and mysterious. Pointing to an iron gate tucked into a corner, he announced: 'The iris garden of Firenze, you must
see it! Is only open two weeks a year!' The *giaggioli* were
captivating. I turned to take his hand but he was already
gone, getting into his car, saying he had a meeting.

'Remember, *amore*,' he called out through the open window as he pulled out into the traffic. 'You are not alone!'

Since my love story had started with Dino, I had not written
a word. I had a good excuse every day but the reality was
that Dino took up most of my time, either being there or
promising to come over, and then sometimes being hours
late or not making it at all. In theory, it shouldn't have mat-
tered as I was just at home writing, but I found that I could
not settle to my work if I was anticipating a visit, from Dino
or anyone else. To sink into the book, I needed an undis-
turbed stretch of time ahead of me, and Dino's habit of
seeming to be always on his way over made me too restless
to concentrate. I resolved to be less available, to prioritise
my routine and rituals and get back to my book.

So it was that the following Saturday morning, I took
an awkward-paced walk to Sant'Ambrogio with my neighbour Giuseppe, taking him first for one of Isidoro's cappuccinos before the market. In Cibreo, I sat down at my
usual seat with Giuseppe opposite.

From the next table, an elderly couple were watching
us. They leant over and greeted Giuseppe. The woman was

small and round, with a dark bob and circular glasses behind which her eyes darted about the room. The man was tall and white-haired, lanky, his long frame draped across the chair. Giuseppe introduced them as Betsy and Geoffrey, American artists, with a house in a village outside Florence where they spent half the year. Betsy told me in an East Coast accent that they had recently arrived for their seasonal stay. They spoke to Giuseppe in Italian, Geoffrey drawling out his words while Betsy's speech was so fast that I couldn't follow. Geoffrey was a painter, Giuseppe explained, while Betsy made ceramics, mostly large pots that Giuseppe told me with a grin were 'wild'.

As they got up to leave Betsy paused by my chair. 'I am just starting a new work and I need a model.' She looked down at me through the fringe of her bobbed hair. 'If you would like to do it, please give me a call. I think you would be perfect.' She handed me a card and I stared after her.

'Well, Giuseppe, shall I do it?' I asked, stunned.

He slowly weighed it up. Then he looked at me and laughed. 'Of course you must do it! It fits with your Florentine adventures, no?' His eyes were twinkling from behind his glasses in a way that made me wonder how much he could actually hear through our walls. 'And she is an important and well-known artist. You will love their house. Now you are so gloriously here, what else can Florence do than immortalise you in art?'

The following evening, Dino was standing in my kitchen, naked apart from an apron tied around his waist. He had just arrived back from a weekend fishing trip in Sicily bearing an ice box and an armful of acacia flowers plucked from the trees outside the city gate. After making love to me on the sofa, he had pulled out two fresh tuna steaks and a jar of Sicilian capers from the ice box. Instructing me to hand him all my fresh tomatoes and garlic, he set about making us dinner.

'*Amore*, this is some of the fish I caught yesterday!' he announced proudly. 'You remember the picture?'

I did indeed. He had neglected to tell me he was going anywhere until the day he was leaving, and at first I had been cross, but in the three days he had been gone, he had bombarded me with pictures of himself in action. Ignoring the poor bleeding fish that co-starred in his pictures, I had focused instead on Dino in his swimming trunks, his body tanned, the muscles bulging as he wrestled the fish, the veins on his arms standing out. He had appeared in one with a knife in his hand, blood running down his biceps. I could forgive him his disappearance if he was going to come back to me laden with fresh fish and in such sporting shape. Now I watched him moving around my kitchen in his porno-chef look, throwing out instructions to me as his sous chef.

'Sit there, *amore*, and talk to me,' he ordered. 'You are much better at talking than cooking.'

I slapped his bare bottom in admonishment and told him about my encounter with Betsy, how nervous I was about accepting the offer of modelling for her.

'I am assuming I would have to be naked,' I shrugged. 'I am not sure I can do it.'

'But why?' he asked.

I blushed. Despite what we had just done, I was shy. 'Well,' I muttered, 'to take my clothes off and have some-one look at me ...'

'But I look at you, *amore*,' he said, 'and you are not ner-vous, you like it.'

'Yes, but that's different,' I cried, 'and anyway you don't really look at me, not at me standing there for hours in detail, do you? I don't exactly have the sort of body that can withstand hours of scrutiny ...'

He stopped cooking to come over and untie the sash on my dressing gown and, holding me at arm's length, looked at me deliberately, slowly. 'Now listen, *amore*,' he said pur-posefully as I squirmed under his gaze. 'You are beautiful and your body is beautiful. You think you are ugly because you are not a supermodel, but you are super you! I love your curves. You look like a woman and that is most beautiful of all.' He planted a kiss in the middle of my chest, on my heart.

'Oh!' I flung my arms around him.

He hugged me back. 'Anyway, *amore*, you don't have to worry,' he said, waving a wooden spoon as I pulled my dressing gown around me, 'if she's nearly eighty, she prob-ably won't be able to see you at all ...'

The evening was relaxed, domestic. The table was deco-rated with flowers from Old Roberto's garden to which we had added the acacia Dino had picked, candles were throw-ing light around the room, the fish was delicious. We were relaxed, at home. I felt so close to him that when, once again after making love to me and falling asleep in my arms, he got up in the dead of night and made for the door, I couldn't bear the crashing disappointment of his departure.

'Dino, why won't you stay?' It was the first time I had allowed myself to ask.

'Because my wife is waiting for me, of course!' he retorted, flaring his nostrils and snorting with derision. I raised my eyebrows and he laughed. Then he paused, saying, 'You think I have time or energy for anyone else, *amore*? You wear me out ...'

I couldn't dispute that. There really seemed no time or energy for another woman. But just to be sure, as I kissed him, I sucked on his bottom lip so hard that I left a bruise, a love bite covering most of his bottom lip, right there on his face, clear for all to see.

'Oh, excuse me, *amore*,' I said, running my finger along the purple stain. 'I got carried away!'

He grinned. 'I love your passion,' he said, kissing me again. 'I don't care who sees it.'

I watched him skipping down the stairs with a wide grin, leaving me vaguely reassured.

I consulted Luigo the next night.

'OK, *bella*, so you are sure he's not married?' he asked, logically.

'Well, I have been known to give him love bites ...' I admitted sheepishly.

Luigo gave me a long look. 'Hickeys, *bella*? How old are we?'

I shrugged. 'I know, but I was suspicious and wanted to know if he would let me.'

'And did he?'

'He positively encouraged me!'

'Has he ever taken you to his place?' Again, Luigo was practical.

'Er, no,' I admitted. 'But that's because he doesn't exactly have his own place.'

Luigo put his tea towel down. 'Are you telling me he lives with his *mamma*?'

Indeed, Dino lived with his parents. At the beginning, he had told me that it was a temporary arrangement, that he had gone to stay there on returning from living in Milan, that he was saving up to buy his own place – the stone house in the country. My shock had been replaced by understanding. 'Ah, OK, that's fair enough.' I too had spent stints at my parents' in between my own flats. 'When did you move back from Milan?'

'Five years ago,' he had replied nonchalantly as my eyebrows shot up.

Luigo nodded. 'He's a *mammone*,' he said. 'Mummy's boys who live at home although they are grown up. Some do it right into their thirties!'

'Oh dear, Luigo, he's forty. That's bad!'

'Well, *bella*, it's quite common here,' he said airily. 'Italian men are very lazy and they love their mamma's cooking, you know. At least we can be sure he's not married. Maybe Mummy gives him a curfew …'

Tuna with capers and tomato sauce

Serves 2

1 white onion
Best-quality extra-virgin olive oil
20 good Sicilian capers

2 cloves garlic
1 400g tin chopped Italian plum tomatoes
Chilli flakes
2 tuna steaks
1 lemon

Chop the onion and fry with olive oil in a pan until translucent, add capers and cook for a short time. Peel and chop the garlic then add. When a little cooked (don't burn), add the tomatoes and let reduce for ten minutes, adding a few chilli flakes.

Cover the tuna steaks in olive oil and squeeze on a lemon, then grill on each side – do not let them become dry. Place on a plate and pour on the tomato sauce. Serve.

Fresh broad bean and pecorino salad

Serves 2

1kg broad beans (as fresh as possible)
150 medium mature pecorino
Juice of 1 lemon

Shell the beans and separate the smaller ones from the larger ones. Pop the large beans into boiling water for just one minute, then drain and put in a bowl of cold water. (I personally don't bother with blanching any of the smaller beans but toss them all in raw.)

Once cooled, peel the outer skin from both the large blanched beans and the small raw ones and throw into a serving bowl. Take the pecorino and cube. Toss in the cheese with the beans. In a small bowl make a pinzimonio dressing (see page 38) with lemon juice, season and whisk. Pour over the salad and toss, then serve.

6

JUNE
Perduta or how to lose your head

Produce in season: watermelon
Scent of the city: jasmine
Italian moment: a Renaissance football match
Italian word of the month: *estate*

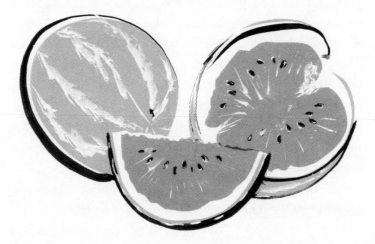

I was practically skipping to the market on Saturday morning. Dino had promised to stay tonight and that meant the whole weekend together. The only time we had spent the whole night together was that turbulent first night in the hotel in Monteriggioni.

I shopped carefully for tomorrow morning's breakfast. Oranges to juice, fresh bread from the *forno*, cherry jam from Cibreo, creamy full-fat milk for our cappuccinos. I filled up on fruit and vegetables and bought packs of fresh pasta in case he wanted to cook at home. I ducked away from Beppe's kisses as I passed Cibreo and walked through the narrow streets leading to the centre smiling at everyone I passed. I called by Pegna to buy a tin of bright yellow butter, only pausing to give Francesca, the humming check-out girl with the sad eyes, a quick hug. Outside the door sweet transcendent voices on the breeze stopped me in my tracks; it was floating over from the back of the Duomo. Francesca joined me on the doorstep, her sad eyes lit up with the beauty of the music as we listened together in silence.

'It's the cathedral choir,' she said in Italian. 'They are practising. One day we sing there together, OK?'

I nodded happily. Walking through the sun-drenched streets dodging the tourists, crossing my ungraceful bridge of graces, looking up at the terraces of the Bardini Gardens that stretched up the slope behind the palazzos, I took a deep breath, trying to inhale it all in – all that beauty, the fresh produce in my bag, the music still ringing in my ears – this place where I lived.

On the way to dinner I had seen a black leather washbag on the back seat of the car and now, strolling back to the flat, Dino was carrying it along with a preternatur- ally giant watermelon that he had bought from a white van parked just outside the city walls. I congratulated myself for my patience and for not being 'insistatious' as he called it.

The scent of flowers and blossoms hit us at the door. '*Amore ma quanto sei carina!*' he cried, spotting the bed I had strewn with rose petals from Old Roberto's garden, the candles all around. I smiled shyly as he lit them.

'Well, you are here. I wanted it to be special.'

We made love, crushing the rose petals under us. Afterwards he got up and sliced some watermelon, pet- als stuck to his moist back, and we sat in bed chatting and eating sweet and juicy fruit. We snuggled up like a real couple. I relaxed against him and snoozed off. So when I woke to see him getting up later, I imagined he was going to the loo – Dino had a penchant for washing himself so fastidiously after sex that I had even bought his penis its own little towel. After this, he had taken to entertaining me by wrapping his penis towel around himself in various styles – a turban, a sailor's cap, even a keffiyeh encircled at the top with one of Christobel's kids' hair elastics.

Now he walked in naked, folding the tiny towel into a mini bandana and placing it over the head of his penis.

'Look, *amore*, doesn't this look just like Stefano, the chef at Nello?'

Stefano was a bald man who wore a white bandana wrapped around his head. Dino's penis did look uncannily like Stefano, and we were both laughing so much that when I saw him picking up his clothes it took me a minute to realise that he was not just arranging them on the chair, but getting dressed.

'*Allora, amore,*' he perched on the edge of the bed from where I regarded him, dumbfounded. 'So now I kiss you and I see you tomorrow.'

'Wait!' My tone startled us both. 'Are you joking? You told me you were staying—'

'*Amore*, no, you are mistaken. I have to go meet a friend now—'

'It's two in the morning, who on earth are you meeting at two in the morning?' My voice was rising.

A story poured out about a friend who had just landed from Paris. Just at that moment, a text pinged on his phone. He made a call and I heard him talking to a male voice which I could hear through the handset. Putting the phone down, he said, 'He just got in from Pisa and now his taxi is bringing him here.'

All the time, he was moving rapidly towards the front door, carrying the washbag. Still naked, I followed him. 'Dino,' I was trying to keep my voice even, 'you said you would stay, you promised. You have seen everything I bought for breakfast ...'

'*Amore*, no. I never promised, *non é possibile* because I was always going to go and see my friend. *Dai*, don't be boring, don't be so *insistatious* ...'

'I don't understand! Look,' I pointed to the washbag clutched in his hand as evidence. 'You brought this. You obviously intended to stay, why have you changed your mind?' What did I do wrong? I wanted to say, but I bit back the words. Fury was beginning to burn through my confusion. He was lying and I couldn't stand it.

'*Amore*, I spend time with my friend now and tomorrow I will be with him, so there is no possibility.' He turned to go, giving me his back, not looking at me as he walked out. 'Go to bed, you are upset and you insist too much. I call you in the morning.'

He ran down the stairs without a backwards glance and I slammed the door so hard that flakes of green paint fell at my feet. Furious, I picked up my phone and stabbed out a message.

this is bullshit u r a liar don't ever come back

I threw myself on the bed and sobbed into the rose petals, all my carefully constructed fantasies of the weekend – of our future together – shattering around me.

'He's scared!' speculated Luigo. 'He knows you will leave and he doesn't want his heart broken.'

Luigo had trotted out his favourite theory every time Dino had called late, cancelled or not stayed the night. I had played along but now I could no longer pretend. I had not heard from Dino for a few days after sending the text, and initially my anger had carried me through, but with uncanny timing, just as I was beginning to miss him, to feel remorseful, he rang me, his tone light and affectionate as if nothing had happened. I had swallowed my questions, my doubts. I had decided to forgive him even though he hadn't apologised.

That night he had been at my door as usual and we hadn't mentioned the other night. I tried to carry on as normal but I now had a more critical perspective of Dino and our 'story'.

I noted Dino's early promises of weekends away exploring Tuscany had never materialised and that our encounters involved him cutting into the routine of my days with promises to come round that weren't always fulfilled. He would find me when I was on one of my long walks and drive me home, make love to me on the sofa and then leave. These appearances left me feeling discombobulated, empty. I was sorry to have my ramblings disturbed only to find myself left again abruptly alone once he had taken his pleasure. I started to wish that we could make proper dates that he would stick to so that I could relish my time alone again. His constant changes and random appearances were beginning to feel like a tyranny. We did have a few evenings together but I was growing tired of being left in the dead of night as he disappeared cheerfully into the dark.

Now I was propping up Luigo's bar alone on a Saturday evening.

'He cancelled again,' I told Luigo, resigned. 'Dinner with some aristocrat he knows from his tennis club. He said it would be rude to say no, he's very influential. And maybe he has a house on his estate in the country that is for rent ...'

Luigo was changing the CD. 'Did he ask you to join him?'

'He did but I said no. He was just being polite, he didn't mean it.'

'Well, *bella*, next time, say yes!' Luigo suggested.

I trailed off to the loo, feeling depressed. Luigo was right. I would call Dino's bluff. I heard Luigo singing along to Duran Duran's 'Rio' in the bar and I dried my hands quickly, cheering up – this song had been the anthem of 1981. I rushed out and landed in the bar just in time to join in with the chorus. We belted it out together, dancing our way around the bar. And we laughed so much that I forgot about Dino for a while.

The next day, I was dressed and waiting for Dino by ten o'clock, looking forward to a day out of the city as promised – my reward for the last-minute cancellation of the night before. Summer was creeping up on us and Florence was heating up, emptying at weekends as the locals headed out to the beach or to the countryside, leaving their city to red-faced tourists. Dino himself had been away the last few weekends, our relationship, I had noticed with dismay, now relegated to weeknights only.

I was excited about the Italian summer. August: the month that the whole country went to the seaside. Dino, I already knew, would take the whole month off. Never had the summer held such allure or been the subject of so many conversations – I heard them every day around the neighbourhood, people planning their August trips, discussing what they would do on the weekend until then. Some of my neighbours had already decamped to *il mare* and I was impressed by how vehemently the Italians believed that time by the sea was their birthright. As a Londoner, the notion of a whole season built around fun, leisure and enjoyment was alien – and deeply seductive too. I thought back to summers past – always working, always alone, always somehow on another deadline even while away. In my mid-thirties it had become harder to find friends to travel with – most were now busy with partners and children and I had found myself going off on impressively glamorous work trips alone.

That summer with Nader had been the first one in years that had contained some of the lightness and joy that summer should have. I had rushed home from work every day, forgetting about the machinations of the Big Boss, the stresses of work, as soon as I walked into my flat. Nader would be waiting for me, sitting on that narrow sofa, smiling, relaxed, a drink prepared. For those three months I'd had someone to come home to. We would go out, wander the streets in the light, long evenings, eat dinner on the pavements of Soho, walk and talk so much we ended up miles away, standing on Waterloo Bridge in front of my favourite view of London.

That Sunday morning Dino was late as usual so I went to Rifrullo, where I sat outside with my mid-morning cappuccino as I waited, battling my irritation. He finally called just before midday. '*Amooorreee*,' he drawled. 'Disaster. I forgot my mother's birthday! Can you imagine? *Mi dispiace*, but I stay home for lunch.'

'Oh, right,' I was deflated.

'Of course you are very welcome to join us,' he said, smooth, fake.

'Oh Dino, well I would love to!' I exclaimed.

'Ah, *amore*, how lovely. I would looovvve that. But you know lunch is all prepared and the guests are all here, I cannot ask them to wait, we are already at the table. And I don't know how you would get here ...'

The excuses rolled off his tongue. So many lies – how could lunch be on the table? It was only midday and Italians never ate so early. But I said nothing. My silence unnerved him.

'*Amore dai*, don't be upset again. I see you later, I always see you, I see you every day.' He was getting defensive, beginning to whine.

I boiled over. 'Actually, Dino, you don't. Every day you say you will come and you don't. And it's OK, you know, I don't need to see you every day. But just make a plan and stick to it,' I snapped. 'Once a week, just say we will have dinner once a week and we'll do that. It's better than hanging around every day waiting for you to turn up. You eat up all my time like this, it's not fair.'

He was taken aback, muttering, 'Well, *amore*, I am like this, if is not OK for you—'

'Yes, well, and I am like this,' I retorted.

'Don't ask me more than I can give, *amore*,' he said quietly. 'I told you how I am.'

'If you can't give me one evening a week, then I guess there's nothing else to say.'

Everyone had heard me shouting – Rifrullo was full of people taking a pre-lunch prosecco – and I decided to march out my fury, to get away from my neighbours and their curiosity. Boiling with anger, each step brought me another realisation of what a fool I had been to believe Dino, to wait for him to stay the night, to form a real relationship.

Hours later I came back, worn out from an epic walk, to find Dino in his car outside my door.

'Where have you been?' He looked cross. 'I have been waiting.'

'How was your lunch?' I asked nonchalantly.

'*Dai amore*,' he took a step forward, '*mi dispiace*, don't be angry,' and he hung his head and opened his arms. 'We go to the country now, I take you, *dai*, is only four, is a beautiful day.'

My head was light and I didn't have the energy to fight. I stepped into the car. We drove out of the gate of San Miniato, the jazzy notes of an Italian song filling the silence. I recognised the word *estate* (summer) in particular. It was beautiful and melancholic, the male voice dripping in nostalgia. Dino turned it up and sang along.

'*Estate*,' he sang in a rich baritone, putting a hand on my knee. I caught only some words that I knew in the melancholy tune which seemed full of longing: '*baci ... perduto ... amore ... passato ... cuore ... cancellare.*' He serenaded me, knitting his brows together for extra drama, his other hand holding a cigarette out of the open window. He steered with his knees. Against my will I felt my mouth twitching into a smile.

When he was finished, he turned to me with a wide grin, waiting for my approbation.

'Well, you have quite a voice,' I said.

'*Amore, si*, at school they called me *il piccolo Pavarotti*!' he said proudly. I chuckled. 'This song,' he explained, 'is one of the greatest Italian songs. Is about a sad love story made in the summer. It says the summer is, you know, full of lost kisses, the love that has passed ...'

I looked at him through narrow eyes. 'Is this prophetic, Dino?' I asked.

'*Amore*, it depends.'

'On what?'

'On this ...' He leant over. '*Baciami, amore!*'

I'd heard this before, I thought, but then all thoughts were blotted out as he pulled over and kissed me so tenderly and for so long that my head started to spin. With some agility, he snapped my seat back so that I was lying down, and with one swift move, he steered his body over mine. I was not quite sure how it happened, parked in a green glade off the road to Chianti, but Dino managed to make swift but forceful love to me in his Audi and I was so surprised that I let him.

Afterwards, we drove through the sun-dappled hills and valleys of Chianti with its mellow stone houses, facades festooned with red geraniums, the sloping hills decorated with olives and vineyards, fields of sunflowers. I pushed away my earlier irritation, my determination to get away from him. It was beautiful, he was sexy and we were here. Perhaps this could be enough.

A few nights later my phone rang. It was Dino from his car on the road to Pisa. He was on his way to Spain for a very fancy wedding, a four-day extravaganza of bullfights and balls. His flight was early the next morning and he was going to stay the night with a friend who lived nearby. At least this is what he had told me.

'*Amore*, don't miss me too much,' he purred down the line. I could hear him dragging on his cigarette, picture his elbow on the open window, the road rushing past. 'On Monday I am in your arms again.'

'I will be patient. Will your phone work there?' I was relaxed; after our evening in the country he had been particularly attentive, coming round to cook every night, spending half the night sleeping with me before leaving, and I had nearly forgotten the spat of the weekend before.

'I call you,' I could hear him smile. 'Or text you. Or I Skype you,' his tone was intimate, reassuring. Then with a flourish: 'Anyway, *amore*, I find a way. If you don't hear from me, you know I am dead!'

'I thought you were dead, *amore*!' exclaimed Antonella sardonically, as she ushered me into the bright interior of her flat.

'*Permesso*,' I said automatically, crossing the threshold and offering up a bouquet of Old Roberto's roses. Antonella took them graciously, burying her nose in their scent, before turning to me with a raised eyebrow.

'Oh Anto,' I cried. 'I am so sorry to have disappeared. I've been so infatuated with Dino ...'

She waved my protests away with an elegant hand. 'Don't speak more of this,' she said sweetly. 'It is good to see you. *La mamma* and I have missed you! Now come through, the Calcio Storico is about to start!'

We filed into her bedroom which was filled with Adonises. She poured me a coffee from a tray already on the table, handing me the china cup and saucer with a tiny silver teaspoon. The Adonises were ranged around the open windows from outside of which came a roar of voices, cheering and calling out, whistling and shouting Florentine obscenities. The Adonises kissed me in turn and parted to let Antonella and I take prime place at each of the windows. It was the last weekend in June and Florence was celebrating the festival of its patron saint, San Giovanni, in spectacular style. The Calcio Storico Fiorentino was an ancient soccer game played out between four of Florence's districts: San Giovanni, Santa Croce, Santo Spirito and Santa Maria Novella. It was taking place in a makeshift stadium that had been constructed over the past week in Piazza Santa Croce, complete with a sand pitch and raised bleachers for the spectators. I knew I was lucky to get to watch from Antonella's window for free – tickets had sold out weeks ago.

The whole city had been in a state of excitement for days. I had bumped into the first procession in anticipation of the Calcio Storico last weekend when, as I returned home from Sant'Ambrogio via the centre on Saturday, I saw men in Renaissance costume parading through the Signoria, some on horses hung with livery, blowing long trumpets and showing off their legs in multicoloured tights. During the week, Antonella had rung to invite me to watch the football match from her window, instructing me to call her from the street so she could walk me through the security barriers – as a resident she was allowed guests.

From early this morning, as soon as I crossed the bridge of graces, I heard the cacophony of Florence happily returning to its Renaissance roots. Last Saturday I hadn't been able to resist pushing my way along the ever-growing crowds on via de Benci to the Signoria to see the tail end of the weekend's parade. As well as the men in their tights and feathered hats, trumpeters with draped flags and liveried horses, there were women holding their long skirts out as they walked, their hair set with diadems, their waists cinched in corsets. It must have been the end as everyone was milling around, talking to friends in regular clothes, peeling off to take a coffee, carefully placing their plumed hats on tables as they smoked.

In Antonella's flat, I leant out and took in the scene. Anto was leaning out of the other window and she called out to me across the gap, raising her voice above the din. Below us were a mass of burly men in Renaissance football shorts – long and shaped a little like knickerbockers, they were baggy and tied at the knee. One team's shorts were striped violet and white while the others were blue and violet. '*Sempre viola*,' shouted Antonella across the windows to me. The Adonis closest to me explained that there had already been two previous matches in which the teams were eliminated down to the two playing today.

'What are the rules, is it like modern football?' I asked him and he laughed.

'Watch, you will see.'

On the night before leaving for Spain, Dino had told me a little about the history of the Calcio Storico. He was cooking a pasta sauce from the fresh young courgettes that were in season with a few slivers of pancetta and a splash of white wine.

'*Amore*, you know of course I am passionate about football?' he started.

I did indeed know that he was a devoted supporter of Florence's football team, Fiorentina, known as the Violas.

'Well, that of course is because we invented football here in Florence!' It was a big claim but he insisted that the tournament had its roots in the sixteenth century, originally played by aristocrats and noblemen.

'It's changed now, most of the guys playing in the teams are convicted criminals ...'

I was intrigued and now, as I looked down at the thickset men who were running around the playing field, covered in tattoos and scars, I could well believe it. There seemed to be hundreds of them on the field at once — the Adonis told me that there were twenty-seven men on each side, and as the game started, there was a scrum more akin to rugby than football. As the game proceeded, the men fell on their opponents, tackling, kicking and even head-butting each other, regardless of whether the ball was in the vicinity. The crowd went wild every time the ball got near the goal but even more so when someone hit someone else — which was often. Despite the best efforts of a referee who ran around waving a big white feather as a sign of his authority, the whole thing degenerated into mass fights several times. I looked at Antonella in shock but she was busy shouting at the players, waving her fist out of the window. All around the square, there were people hanging out of windows and on balconies, shouting and gesticulating wildly. Even *la mamma*, who had popped her head out to check on the match's progress, was shouting

something, her hands cupped around her mouth. The
Adonises were all transfixed, mostly watching the muscles
ripple on the brawny bodies on the pitch, and the crowd
was almost as out of control as the players, having argu-
ments and fist fights among themselves in the bleachers.

I started to laugh. Giuseppe had once told me that the
great puzzle of the Renaissance was how such refined art
and architecture could have been produced by people
who were essentially as rough and violent as street thugs.
Dino's own belligerence and love of dominance could, I
imagined, quickly turn to aggression and indeed I could
clearly see him in my mind's eye stalking the streets of
sixteenth-century Florence, his small taut body in tights,
ruffled shorts and feathers, his sword poised and ready to
run through an enemy as he crossed the Ponte Vecchio. I
looked down again at the spectacle of flouncy costumes
and hulking muscles, feathers trodden into the sand, the
iris-bearing flag of Florence flapping around the bleachers,
the crowd shouting obscenities, and wondered if anything
had really changed in Florence in the past five centuries
apart from the outfits.

Later, we stood on the banks of the Arno in crowds that
included all my San Niccolò neighbours, watching fireworks burst over the sky above San Miniato. The display
was the climax of the festival of San Giovanni and it illuminated the city, lit up the river. It was beautiful. The heat
of the day had simmered down to a balmy still evening. I
wished Dino was here, and I instinctively pulled out my
phone to check if he had rung. He had been gone two days

and there'd been no word of him. I found this odd, but I told myself that he was in Spain, busy with his friends, and perhaps there was no reception. That I would hear from him soon; that, as he had assured me with his parting words, he would always find a way to communicate. I took a photo of the fireworks exploding in the dark sky with my phone and sent it to him, expecting to hear from him as soon as it went through, but there was no call and no answering text. I saw Antonella watching me and gave her a watery smile.

'He'll ring soon, don't worry,' she said kindly, and took my hand in hers.

I nodded, watching fire explode in the sky. But worry gnawed at me and, for the first time in all these months in Florence, I couldn't give myself over completely to enjoying its beauty.

Pasta with courgettes

Serves 2

2 courgettes
1 white onion
Best-quality extra-virgin olive oil
1 clove garlic
Sea salt, to taste
150–200g pasta (I like penne)
½ glass white wine
Parmesan, to serve

Top and tail the courgettes and cut them lengthways into two. Then slice. Chop the onion and fry in a pan with olive oil until translucent. Chop the garlic and add to the pan. Cook a little then add the courgettes along with a splash of water – a couple of tablespoons will do.

At the same time, fill a large pasta pot with water and, when it is boiling, add salt. Add the pasta, and cook till al dente. Add some of the pasta water to the courgettes, and the white wine.

When the courgettes are cooked but still moist, drain the pasta and add to the pan till the sauce covers all, then grate on some Parmesan. Serve.

Wild rocket and Parmesan salad

Serves 2

Two handfuls fresh wild rocket
Mature Parmesan
Juice of 1 lemon
Sea salt and black pepper, to taste

Wash the rocket carefully and let it dry, then add some long, fine slivers of Parmesan. Make a pinzimonio (see page 38) with lemon juice, season liberally with salt and black pepper, and pour over the salad, tossing it all together. Serve.

7

JULY
Piacere a te stessa or how to take
pleasure in yourself

Produce in season: San Marzano tomatoes
Scent of the city: roses
Italian moment: a visit to the beauty salon
Italian word: *brillare (to sparkle)*

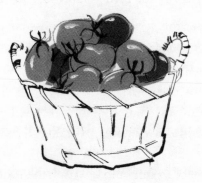

I was on one of the little yellow buses rumbling out of the city, heading to Bagno a Ripoli, a small town to the south of Florence. It was the day after the Calcio Storico, the date long arranged for the start of my modelling career, and I was going to a tiny hamlet where Betsy and Geoffrey lived.

In preparation, I had shaved my legs carefully and regarded myself in the mirror, sucking in my tummy, choosing good underwear, massaging cream into my body. It was a welcome distraction from waiting for Dino to ring – it was the Sunday morning of his trip to Spain and still I had not heard from him. Betsy had told me to bring a swimsuit and I had picked up the only bikini I could find in the market, mortifying as it was – I usually tried to hide as much of my body as possible in a swimsuit but my budget made buying a one-piece from one of the boutiques in the centre prohibitive. For the first time in years, I would wear a bikini. Trying it on at home later, I had blushed. And yet, as I turned and examined my body from every angle, I couldn't deny that it actually looked OK. More than OK, it was almost slim, just the hint of one roll left on my back instead of the three I had arrived with. Still, I hoped that there would be no one but Betsy at the pool with me.

Betsy met me in the village piazza wearing a stripy summer dress with green plimsolls and pink ankle socks. She was voluble and colourful, full of exuberant curiosity as

she drove us into the wooded hills, a rough road leading
to a cluster of houses clinging to a steep slope. There were
only six houses here, she told me, made up of two families. She and Geoffrey had bought their house forty years
ago, and they were now part of this small community.
'Although,' she said with a wink, 'it took a few years ...'

We stepped through metal gates painted blue, the high
stone walls closing the house off from the street. Inside,
there was a courtyard and a shaded terrace that looked
out over a deep valley, a stone table and benches set with
Betsy's pottery. At the back of the house there was another
nook hanging out over the valley into which was built a
round table, and I sat here while Betsy made us coffee. I
looked down over the countryside falling away all around
me and spotted the dome of Florence's cathedral far in
the distance, tiny. The air was warm and still, the day alive
with the noises of the country, the chirping of birds, the
chirruping of insects, the hum of bees. There were pigeons
and turtle doves fluttering around an aviary that occupied
the other side of the courtyard and, at my feet, I spotted a
small tortoise with an exquisite shell.

Betsy arrived with our coffees and, after setting them
down, went and opened the door of the aviary. The birds
flew out, the doves flapping above our heads before they
disappeared into the valley, a few loose feathers floating
down. I felt a nip on my big toe and looked down to see
the tortoise nibbling on my nail. 'Oh, ignore him,' Betsy
said, laughing, 'he'll stop in a moment.' For the first time
all weekend, I relaxed and enjoyed myself, happy to talk to
Betsy about her life, her art, about my book. That morning

with Betsy brought me back to myself, reminded me
that there was more to me than this story with Dino. She
quizzed me about the themes of the book, talked of process
and patience, of a lifetime of creating. And I found myself
confiding in her about Dino – his sporadic reliability, how
I hadn't heard from him for a few days. Her intelligent eyes
regarded me from behind her thick glasses.

'Ah, Italian men,' she laughed. 'They are a law unto
themselves. But,' with a twinkle, 'so delightful. Every girl
should have an Italian romance. Remind me to tell you a
story from my youth later. Now, let's get to work.'

She led me down the path into the garden. The main
house was supplemented by both her and Geoffrey's studios, each occupying a different terrace cut into the hill,
stone dining areas and lounges built out over the drop into
the valley. Everywhere there were statues and benches
built by Betsy, large pots she had made as well as their
own attempt at *sgraffito* etched on the walls. Her studio
was several terraces down with a large kiln outside, the
bright green lawn in front dug up with what looked like
small tractor tracks. 'Wild boar,' she explained, indicating
them. 'They sometimes come in from the woods and run
rampage here, they destroy the grass.'

'Aren't you scared?' Dino would love this, I thought. He
could come hunting here.

She laughed. 'No, they never come when there are
people around. They are shy, magnificent creatures. Now,'
opening the door, 'come in.'

Betsy's studio was large and light, one side covered in
sliding French doors. Trestle tables lined the walls and

stood arranged at regular intervals through the room. Some walls bore cubbyholes filled with pigments, paints, brushes. Elsewhere there was a potter's wheel and sacks of powder, sketchbooks and, leaning against the walls, giant ceramic works that defied description. Neither pots nor sculptures, they were like giant ceramic paintings with jagged edges and fins sticking out. In contrast to their challenging forms they were painted in happy colours, with squiggles that resembled flowers or vases, reminiscent of Matisse. In the middle of the room were her other works, the pots she was famous for, standing tall, their shapes conforming to nothing I had seen. Betsy explained when they had been made, what had inspired her. As I picked my way carefully through this ceramic wonderland, I realised what a privilege it was to be here in her studio, examining pieces at such close quarters that were usually only visible in the museums and galleries of the world, with the artist herself explaining them to me. I shuddered to think how stupid I had been, letting my life be reduced to Dino and his whims. This was why I was here – to create – and Betsy's studio inspired me to refocus on the main purpose of my life.

'Now,' she turned to me. 'As you can see, I never decorate my pots with human figures. I have a work now that has been puzzling me for some time but when I met you in Cibreo that time, something clicked.' She laughed. 'You reminded me of it. That's why I asked you to model for me!'

I reminded you of a pot? I wanted to say, instinctively sucking in my belly, but Betsy explained as she led me to a corner of the studio. 'It's a triptych that works together, they complete each other …'

And she indicated three large white pots. But to call them pots would be to call Botticelli's *Venus* a sketch. They were as much sculptures in ceramics as anything else. Two were as tall as me, and in the middle there was one that was long, slim, curvaceous like a female form. They were white and undecorated but placed next to each other like that, with fins and broad flat handles extending out, they completed each other, the spaces between them as much a part of them as their geometric protrusions. The positive and negative forms worked together to make a vibrant whole. And none of them were wide-bellied pots as I had imagined when Betsy told me I somehow reminded her of them – they were slender, lissom even, and there was something undoubtedly feminine about them. I was flattered.

Betsy handed me a dressing gown, and as I went behind a screen to undress, she went on talking. 'This is the first time I have used the human form, I am quite nervous!' and she giggled. I came out to find her arranging her paints and brushes behind the works. She indicated where I should stand, and I slowly took off the dressing gown, throwing it over a nearby ladder, standing awkwardly with my arms crossed. Betsy ignored my self-consciousness and applied herself with no-nonsense practicality to helping me find the right pose. She made shapes with her small round body, trying out the poses herself until we found a position that worked. I shifted my weight from foot to foot, trying to find a comfortable position, still unable quite to look Betsy in the eye.

'Don't worry,' she said in her East Coast drawl. 'This is really a sketch, you don't have to stand perfectly still. I just need a kind of outline ...' She measured her perspective, holding out a paintbrush, her attention more on her pots and the lines she was painting on them than on my body. I started to relax as she told me of her life with Geoffrey, how they divided their time between Tuscany and New York, saying: 'You know, I love New York. But it's much too stimulating to create art. That's why we spend six months a year here. Apart from how beautiful this house is, it's just so nice to let the mind be washed clean of all that over-stimulation. After a month or so here, I am ready to create again – that's why I didn't ask you before now.' Indeed, it had been more than a month since we had first met. She went on: 'I'm a child of the city, I couldn't stay here all the time, but as an artist, the city exhausts me. Here in Tuscany, with its amazing light and landscape and art, I fill right back up. I can slow down. And this laziness in the lifestyle here – I find it very conducive to creativity.' For the first time she looked me in the eye. 'I expect you find the same thing? With your writing?'

It had been a while since I had occupied that peaceful space in which I walked and visited art and wrote. But now I saw that she was right. In the first months after arriving, it was as if the stresses of London had drained out of me and Florence had soaked in instead, marinating my burnt-out brain in beauty. The laziness had lulled me, allowed my thoughts to expand, words to come up unbidden. Dino and the heart-thumping excitement created by his presence had put a stop to that. The sense I always had that he might not show up, that he was dangerous – it upset the delicate balance of peace and stimulation that had enabled me to write. Betsy was the first person to talk to me as an artist, and I liked this reflection of myself. I was so lost in thought that I forgot I was naked. Betsy's gaze, as she stood behind her pots, was impersonal – she was in her own world now – and a peaceful silence descended.

It didn't take long. An hour and three poses later, Betsy had sketched my form out in thick paint on the three pots. She beckoned me over and I looked at them, loose outlines of full breasts, a bellybutton, a swell of buttocks, all topped off by a headful of big curls. There were no details and yet it was me. And it was beautiful. I turned and, impulsively, threw my arms around her. She hugged me back. We looked at each other and smiled wordlessly. She knew as well as I did what I meant. And then I laughed, embarrassed, as I realised I was still naked.

'Come on,' she said brightly, 'let's have a swim before lunch! That was a good morning's work.' I donned my bikini, no longer mortified by it, and we dipped in the infinity pool built out on a ledge overlooking the valley, the water spilling over the sides of the pool into the horizon. Afterwards I helped Betsy carry out to the long stone table plates of cold roast vegetables, salad, chunks of bread and oil, a *tricolore* of creamy buffalo mozzarella sliced with tomatoes and fat leaves of basil. She cut us half-moon slices of very sweet watermelon and made us coffee. And before driving me back down to the village piazza and the bus, she pressed a hundred euros on me. 'This is how much Geoffrey always pays his models. I hope it's enough?'

'Betsy, no!' I cried. 'I am not a model, you mustn't pay me!'

But she insisted. 'You have given me your day and your body to transform my work. Of course I must pay you. Your time has value, you know.'

I dozed on the bus, my phone clutched in my hand. It had been a lovely day and Betsy had made posing for her easy, companionable. I had rarely felt so comfortable in my body. It was a golden interlude before the dark days that followed.

Dino never did ring. Not that night, not that weekend, not ever. I never heard from him again. Just like that, Dino went to Spain and disappeared from my life. Had he vanished in a cloud of smoke in front of my eyes it couldn't have been more mysterious or surprising.

That first weekend felt like the longest of my life. Back from Betsy's, I paced about my flat for the rest of the day, chewing my nails. I didn't know what to do with myself, so unmoored was I by his silence. So I went to see Luigo on Monday as soon as he arrived for work.

'Luigo, what if something has happened to him?' I asked feverishly. 'I mean, he should have landed a couple of hours ago, he should be back in Florence, but I have tried ringing him and his phone is still off.'

Luigo regarded me calmly. 'Any minute, *bella*, he will call!' he said with confidence. 'You know what a flake he is, he probably left his phone somewhere ...'

'Yes, but once when I rang it rang, and then it was off, so I was thinking perhaps he had left it somewhere and it had run out of charge but then it rang and rang again and that's not possible if it has been left in a room in Pisa, say ...'

I heard myself ranting, but I couldn't stop. I couldn't imagine any possible reason other than illness or death that would have prevented Dino from being in touch with me for four days. Since meeting three months ago, we had never gone so long without talking or sending a message. It was inexplicable.

But the week lumbered on with no word from Dino, and I began to realise there would be none. The three-month anniversary of our first kiss, our first date, our first (and only) night together came and went and there was still no word, not a peep, a message, a text. As if to make things worse, with the arrival of July a stultifying humidity descended on Florence. Every time I walked out of my building, a wave of hot air heavy with moisture hit me in the face. People disappeared from the streets during the heat of the day, and I had to stop my walks after I came home one day with sunstroke, vomiting for a whole afternoon, lying on the cool bathroom floor my phone still gripped in my hand. I had sent a pathetic text to Dino then, saying: I'm sick. Help? sure that he wouldn't be able to resist, he had always been so solicitous. I resolved that if he rang then I would say nothing of his disappearance, would forgive him, do all I could to go back to the way things were. But there was no response.

The flat was not much better than the streets; the heat sat heavy. I found a small fan in the cupboard off the hall

but it barely alleviated the heat. I didn't have air-condi-
tioning, and nor did Rifrullo or Luigo's either. I couldn't
walk across town to the market or Cibreo. I learnt to close
my shutters as the Florentines did, to shut out the sun, and
the dark muggy air depressed me further.

The following Friday night I was at Luigo's. He had
opened a terrace outside the bar, put a handful of tables on
the street under an awning. We sat there, fanning ourselves
as he dragged on a cigarette and I chewed on the last nail
that I had not already bitten to the quick. I had also chewed
Luigo's head off all week and I still had no other topic of
conversation. And yet he listened patiently. 'Even if he
extended his trip for some reason, he should be back from
Spain by now, how can he not call me or take my calls?
There must be something wrong. His Skype is switched
off too.' I still couldn't quite believe his disappearance had
anything to do with not wanting to see me. He had had
bursts of unreliability before but never for so long and
over all possible modes of communication. 'Luigo,' I said
seriously. 'What if he's dead?'

'*Bella*, he's not dead, *dai*,' Luigo reasoned. 'You'd know
if he was, someone would tell you.'

'Would they?' I demanded. 'Who would tell me? I don't
know his friends and his family ...'

'You met lots of his friends, didn't you?' Luigo was
right, we had been joined at Nello by plenty of people, but
I didn't know them beyond their first names. I didn't have
anyone's phone number. I had never been to his home, met
his family; in fact, I didn't even know where he lived. How
had I never noticed any of this before?

Nothing else occupied my overheated brain all week, in spite of the promise I had made to myself at Betsy's to return to my writing routine. It dawned on me that Dino had treated me like an affair. Always coming to my flat or taking me out of town in the evenings. He had revealed nothing about himself. The reality now hit me like a train. Our relationship, no matter how romantic and close it had felt to me, added up to very little of substance. All I had imagined between us melted away, the future I had written for us deleted to nothing. I was in shock.

But he had behaved as if he had nothing to hide. When he checked his email from my computer, he saved his password and never logged out. And so it was that one night, desperate for some contact, feeling half crazy in the heat, I decided to check his email. That way, I could at least see if he was picking up mail – proof that he was alive. I opened his web browser and clicked into his inbox, pushing aside my misgivings at this invasion of his privacy, finally feeling calmer to be taking some action.

The email I had sent him had been opened. He had been online. Instant relief. A quick look at his sent box revealed that he had been writing emails the day before. They were short, hurried – he'd probably only been online for ten minutes – but nonetheless, there were no emails to me.

The relief that he was OK was quickly followed by outrage – how could he be alive and not call me? A few days ago we had been together, close, in love, I was his *amore*. And now he was avoiding my calls, hiding on Skype, ignoring me. Just like that, from one day to the next, he had erased me from his life. Only now did I realise that although I had made him the centre of mine, I had actually not been part of his life at all.

I was sprawled like a starfish across the double bed, naked. The window was open and the fan sat on the rickety table in front of me. A salty film of sweat covered my body, my iPod was playing 'Estate' on a loop. I knew the words by heart by now and I sang along, silent tears running down my face. Every word could have been written for me: 'summer, which gave its perfume to each flower, the summer which created our love, only then to make me die of pain ...'

The summer was, indeed, killing me. The season that had promised so much had me prone, useless, unable to do anything but lie around and cry. I never knew I could sweat so much.

When I was not crying, I was furious. In the days since breaking into his email for the first time, my anger had burnt hotter than the scorching midday sun. Hacking into his email had become an obsession. I had recruited Kicca to translate his emails but trawl as we might through mails and pictures that friends had sent of the wedding in Spain (Dino looking handsome in a morning suit, Dino playing the fool in a bullring, Dino in a line of tall, besuited men), rake as my eyes did his face for any clue to his state of mind, we had found no smoking gun.

The heat rose up all day, reaching me at the top of the building with such ferocity that in the middle of the afternoon I had to switch off my computer to stop it overheating and lie in a cold bath. I now understood why people escaped the city on the weekends for the fresh breezes of the coast, but I had no choice. Weekends of messing about on boats with Dino remained a distant dream, although his emails and their attached pictures showed me that he was busy with jaunts: a weekend in Sicily (in linen dancing on a beach at twilight), a fishing trip to Sardinia (action shots grappling with fish), a chic party in St Tropez (going up the steps of a private plane) and a walk in the sea with a prominent female politician at an upscale beach resort: he had been papped walking thigh-high in the surf with her, his sunglasses on, a new moustache decorating his top lip, almost unrecognisable.

My weekends were empty. I was lost; he had rung five times a day, his habit of seeming always on his way had filled my days. Now that I had been dumped out into the dull reality of normal life, I had no routine to ground me, nothing to save me from thinking. Motivating myself to sit in front of my computer and push on with the book was impossible. I dreaded going out into my street. We had been such a public couple and now I couldn't face everyone, their curiosity, their kindness. I slunk out in the early evenings, up to the hills, where I watched well-dressed couples coming home, stepping elegantly into their villas, and felt locked out of this chic domesticity. The city that had opened its arms to me now felt alien and impenetrable, governed by rules I didn't understand.

I want my mum, I thought feverishly one day as I lay curled up on the corner sofa. I rang her crying and in a move so unexpected that it roused me out off the sofa to start

cleaning again, my mother announced she was coming to
see me. Coming to get me was what she implied. I snapped
into action.

My parents, while always supportive, had never really
recovered from my refusal to continue living with them
– like a good Iranian girl – until I was married. Straight
after university I had moved in with friends, and while
they accepted my British insistence on independence,
they rarely came to visit me in my own flats; I always went
home to them.

Now, my mother was coming to take care of me, and
I was so surprised that I battled the heat to visit the market, filling my fridge with the plenty of summer – deep
red San Marzano plum tomatoes, small courgettes with
their trumpet-like flowers, sweet plums and burgundy
mulberries that stained my fingers.

A few days later she was in my flat, pulling from her
suitcase packets of basmati rice, dried barberries, jars of
Iranian pickles carefully swaddled in bubble wrap, pots of
Persian saffron and turmeric. Despite my protestations that
there was food in Italy, she had come to my rescue with the
tools for the type of healing she excelled at – her cooking.

My mother's kitchen has always been my haven, an
Iranian oasis in the desert of dull English food. Smelling
of herbs and spices, it was a place of permanent culinary
activity: chopping parsley, cleaning coriander, grinding the
dark orange threads of saffron into a vivid powder, rice
bubbling in water on the cooker. Yet, despite her passion
for cooking and the refinement of her presentation – rice
sprinkled with shards of cut pistachios and orange peel,

pink dried rose petals scattered over homemade yoghurt – she could not pass her skills on. A perfectionist by nature, and a society hostess by training, my mother could not countenance a tomato cut badly, a lettuce shredded the wrong way, and my clumsiness and impatience brought us to loggerheads. I had retired from any attempt at cooking a long time ago, but had never lost the taste for my mother's food, its bountiful flavours carrying the memories of Iran and my childhood.

Our first stop was the market. By now I had found a way to get across the city in the heat. I skirted the palazzos on the sides of the streets, pausing by their basement windows – which opened to the street at pavement level – to cool my ankles in the fresh air that came blowing out. Now I led my mother to the market, teaching her how to stick close to the buildings, walking in the shade of their wide roofs, and we scuttled across the city like a couple of shy mice.

My mother loved the market and worked her way through the stalls like the old hand that she was. When we had first arrived in London, at the tail end of the drab 1970s, the supermarkets had been a sad affair and the paucity of English fruit distressed her. At first she had taken refuge in Harrods' food hall, the Iranian diaspora's default setting in those days – when in doubt, head to Harrods – but she had eventually found her way to both Portobello and Church Street markets, filling up there on the large bunches of herbs and piles of fruit and vegetables we had been used to in Iran. Now I led her to Antonio's stall, where he took her hand and bent so low over it in greeting that I worried he would fall. Like two old friends, they busied themselves, my mother pointing to the produce she wanted, rejecting anything Antonio picked up that she didn't like the look of. Unlike his bossy way with me, with my mother Antonio was acquiescent and respectful, keeping his place in the face of a superior authority. They got on famously despite having no common language, and I was sure that somehow, in the middle of their inexplicable communication, they even laughed at me and my shopping habits.

Back home she got to work straight away, and before long pots were bubbling on the stove, tomatoes being turned into paste, the smell of saffron rising from the rice as she stained it expertly. It wasn't until we sat down to eat a delicious and comforting Persian meal that I finally confided in her, told her about Dino and his disappearance.

Had I not been so desperate, I would have said nothing. Although we were close in our way, I was still the typical immigrant child, keeping the English part of my life – with its sex and myriad modern problems – to myself, presenting my parents instead with an idealised version of myself. Through the painful years of the Big Job, I had hidden the extent of my distress from them, even while its physical manifestations were plain for all to see. But now, Dino's desertion had me floored and I could not – did not want to – hide it from my mother. My tears dripped into the steam rising from my rice and aubergine stew. When I finished telling her everything, my mother reached out and took my hand. 'You know why you are crying, *azizam*?' she asked softly. 'It's not so much for that man really. It's because of the death of the fantasy. That's much harder to let go of, you know. Reality,' she sighed, 'well, real love is messy and uncomfortable and challenging. But it's so much better, you'll see.'

I was trailing Antonella through town after putting my mother on the train to the airport. I had cried saying good-bye to her, and we had hugged tight. It had been a short trip but rich with comfort and closeness. We had gone to the market every day, had been delighted to discover it full of sour cherries, and had taken a whole box home in a taxi, where, after an hour of washing then patiently pitting each cherry, my mother showed me her method for making my childhood favourite, sour cherry jam. From a little of its dark thick syrup she had made me a *sharbat*, the traditional Iranian fruit syrup mixed with a little water and lots of ice to beat the heat, and put the rest in my fridge for the following days. She had taught me how to make my own yoghurt, inspired by the creamy milk from the Maremma, showing me how to strain it through muslin to make it thick and tangy. She had packed my freezer with her rich tomato-based Persian stews, had tucked the packets of basmati rice into my cupboards, and with that, she had departed, leaving me with the tastes of my homeland as solace.

Antonella was on her way to the hairdresser and I fol-lowed her into the salon, entering a world of noisy, female banter. She introduced me to Maria, the salon owner, a wild-haired older woman who settled in with us after bringing us coffee, and as another woman attended to colouring Antonella's locks, talk turned – as it does in such settings the world over – to men and our love lives. I explained, through Antonella, what had just happened with Dino. To my surprise, instead of being shocked, Maria and the attendant women all nodded sagely.

'*Eh*,' said a stately woman from under a hood hairdryer. 'It's happened also to me ...'

'Me too,' piped up a young woman from the other chair, her hair wrapped in foil. '*Sono stronzi!*'

Antonella turned to me: 'You see, *bella*, you're not alone.'

Maria cupped one of my cheeks in her hand. 'These *stronzi* happen to us all,' she said kindly. 'You mustn't take it personally, a beautiful girl like you.'

I did take it personally. I found it impossible to separate Dino's behaviour from myself, my looks. 'I feel so ugly,' I wailed and Maria exchanged a glance with Antonella.

'*Guarda, bella*,' said Maria. 'I have an idea. You have beautiful hair,' she stroked my head tenderly. 'Have you ever thought about wearing it shorter?'

'Cut that man right out of your hair, *tesoro*,' nodded Antonella.

I hesitated. My hair had been this length for as long as I could remember. But in this heat, I felt nothing but the dead weight of all those curls, crowding around me as I lay unsleeping in bed at night. Now, as I looked at Maria, I nodded my assent. Why not, I thought, cut that bastard out of my hair?

Maria prepared her scissors as I had my hair washed, the whole salon joining in with ideas. But Maria had her own plan. And as I sat down next to Antonella, Maria's scissors flew round my head, snipping and cutting, a mass of black curls tumbling to the floor.

'It's like a black sheep is being shorn, *cara*,' laughed Antonella. I looked at Maria anxiously and she gave me a reassuring pat on the shoulder. 'Don't worry,' she said, 'is going to be perfect. I was thinking – do you know Gina Lollobrigida …?'

I smiled, and even more broadly when Maria had finished, putting down her hairdryer and turning my chair to face the whole salon. A cheer went up from the women, choruses of '*ma dai, che bella!*' When Maria turned my chair to face the mirror, I was dumbstruck. She had transformed me into a 1950s starlet, given me a head of curls that sat as glamorously as if on Ava Gardner.

'*Guarda*,' said Antonella proudly. 'You are the Iranian Sophia Loren. *Bellissima!*'

'"*Ogni donna puo figurare al meglio se sta bene dentro la proprio pelle*,"' recited the woman from under the humming hood. '"*Non c'entrano i vestiti ed il trucco, ma come si brilla.*" *Ha detto la grande Sophia …*'

Antonella translated: 'Every woman can appear her best if she stays well inside her own skin. Clothes and make-up don't matter, it's how you shine …'

'*Sante parole*,' nodded the other woman sagely.

I hugged Maria. 'Listen,' she said, 'forget that *stronzo* and listen to me. *Impara a piacere a te stessa.*' I looked at her blankly.

'It's Latin,' said Antonella. 'From Seneca. It means something like "learn to take pleasure at yourself". Is the same like say La Loren.'

'Be pleased with myself?' I asked. They nodded furiously. I embraced everyone in the salon and, walking home, I paused once or twice to gaze at my reflection in the shop windows, taking pleasure in myself.

That night, I went to the Boboli Gardens to meet Betsy. I had tickets to see an open-air opera which I had booked for me and Dino. I had invited Betsy instead and I found her waiting for me with blankets and mosquito repellent. I showed her my new hairstyle proudly and she complimented me as enthusiastically as an Italian. 'You know who it reminds me of? Do you know Gina Lollobrigida?' and I laughed.

As we sat down and started rubbing the chemicals into our bare ankles, I told Betsy the story of Dino's disappearance. She paused in her ministrations and looked at me with an impish smile. 'Oh yes, I am not surprised,' she said. 'Italian men don't change. I had the exact same thing happen to me fifty years ago right here in Florence.'

'Do you think it was his father?' I said, and we laughed our heads off.

We swapped stories of our love affairs, howling at all the similarities, the half century stretching between them notwithstanding. 'You see,' she said to me in between rapid-fire bursts of laughter, 'getting your heart broken by a rogue Italian man is part of the education, my dear. Don't let it put you off Italy. Look, I am still here fifty years later. There's a lot more for you here in Florence than this shifty Dino.'

Sour cherry jam

Makes 1 jar

3 cups sour cherries
1 cup white sugar

Wash and pit the cherries, and cut them into halves. Cover in sugar and leave to sit for as long as you can – at least a couple of hours, overnight if possible.

Boil in a deep pan over a medium-high heat, stirring constantly. After 10 minutes, pour out some of the excess syrup, which you can keep in the fridge and dilute with water and drink with plenty of ice – a super-refreshing *sharbat*. Carry on cooking the cherries. Do not overcook; you can judge by the depth of the red colour – not too dark, probably another 5 minutes.

Sterilise a jam jar. Pour in the jam and, once cooled, refrigerate. Because there is no pectin, this will keep in the fridge for only 2–3 weeks, so eat within that time.

Natural yoghurt

2 litres full-fat milk
4 tsp live natural yoghurt

Pour the milk into a large pan and bring to the boil, stirring constantly – this way it stays at boiling point for longer and becomes more creamy. Remove immediately – you don't want it to burn.

Pour into a large ceramic bowl and allow it to cool until the sides of the bowl are just comfortably warm – a little warmer than tepid. This takes time, so be patient.

Carefully mix the yoghurt into the milk, making sure the yoghurt is not too cold. Take a towel and cover the bowl, wrapping it all the way round (I first place a cloth of muslin on top, allowing the muslin to gently touch the surface of the milk). Leave in a warm place for between 6–8 hours (the longer you leave it, the tarter it will become. I prefer my yoghurt relatively tart – the Iranian way – so I leave it overnight). Then unwrap your yoghurt which should be beautifully set – the muslin will have absorbed the water, but any remaining water can be spooned off (drink this, it's super-good for you!). Put in the fridge for at least a couple of hours, then it's ready to eat. It will keep for at least a week.

8

AUGUST
Femminilità or how style has nothing to do with money

Produce in season: white peaches and mulberries
Scent of the city: sewers
Italian moment: drinking wine on the street at twilight
Italian word of the month: *silenzio*

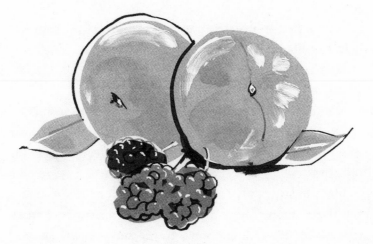

On the first day of the month, I met Antonella at a tiny café inside Sant'Ambrogio's covered market. Cibreo was closed and this was the only place still open nearby. It was sweltering hot and I was in a pair of shorts and a spaghetti strap top, flip-flops on my feet – I knew I had failed spectacularly to make *la bella figura*. Antonella was wearing a black structured sundress, accessorised with pointy pumps and red lipstick. Her hair was pulled back into a low ponytail. She was cool, elegant and a little edgy. She looked me up and down, the customary Italian flick of assessment, bold and unashamed. I stood under her gaze, put my arms out a little and twirled around for good measure.

'I look like an American tourist, I know,' I pre-empted her. 'I apologise. But it's hot.'

'Darling, you do,' she drawled. 'But I love you so I forgive you.'

'I'm also skint and I have nothing else for this heat.'

'No problem, *cara*. On Sunday come to the Pulci with me, I introduce you to my vintage man before he goes on holidays.'

On Sunday, I duly turned up at the Mercato dei Pulci, the flea market. Today there was also a bric-a-brac market, makeshift stalls spilling into the surrounding streets. Antonella was waiting for me on one side of the square, wearing the biggest sunglasses I'd ever seen. She was standing next to a rickety stall piled high with a jumble of clothes. Alongside there were two rails of dresses, hanging dangerously close to her burning cigarette. She gestured me over and introduced the grizzled-looking man behind the stall as Alessandro, saying he had the best vintage gear and the best prices. I looked at Alessandro dragging hungrily on a cigarette stub; he looked like he had come straight from a party.

'Alessandro is a DJ!' said Antonella, pawing through a pile of clothes. 'Darling,' she fixed me with a red-rimmed eye over the top of her humongous sunglasses, 'I left the party last night at three and he was still there ...'

He really had come straight from a party. Alessandro turned a toothless grin on me – alcohol seeped from his sweat – and let loose a rapid fire of broad Tuscan. I turned to Antonella to translate but she was too busy pulling out unpromising-looking rags which, after a vigorous shake from her, turned out to be quirky fashion items from past decades. More than an eye, Anto was possessed of a laser-guided fashion radar capable of honing in on a stray piece of rare Issey Miyake or 1980s Moschino hiding at the bottom of a pile of crap even with a hangover that rendered her practically blind. She was a marvel and she was on my side. She helped me find an armful of pieces – a soft cotton top here, a pair of pleated 1980s shorts there. I left with two tops, the shorts, a T-shirt and a pair of trousers, all for fifty euros, and felt very pleased with myself. No more cringing around town looking like a tourist, I could now waft through the piazzas in my linen palazzo pants, stay cool and look stylish. Antonella's last act was to take

pity on my feet. 'Are you on the beach?' she said pointedly, arching a brow at my flip-flops. So I let her steer me
towards a pair of old Chanel ballet pumps, beige with a
half-moon of black at the tip. 'Vintage, darling, not old,'
she corrected me. 'Sandals are not a good idea in the city
for so many reasons. Florence is dirty, *cara*, there is dog
poo everywhere, so closed shoes are best for the day. You
can show off your pedicure at the beach.'

'I'm not going to the beach,' I sighed. 'I'm British, we
don't do that. We work in August.'

'I know, I know. But anyway, wear your pretty sandals
at night, when some handsome guy is driving you around.'

'I will never date again, Antonella. Especially not an
Italian man! No more lifts in Audis. From now on I have
to walk everywhere by myself, so I suppose the pumps are
practical ...'

Walking home later, thrilled with my purchases, it
struck me that Antonella had expertly nudged me out of
my casual dressing habits and shared her jealously guarded
vintage dealer, outfitting me for the summer at a fraction
of the sum I would have spent on a pair of shoes in my
former life. She had made me recall the sight of filthy feet
in flip-flops on the Tube in London in the summer, giving
me the gift of elegance, teaching me how to take pride in
my appearance, whatever my budget or my mood. I had
never seen Antonella out without her red lipstick on and
I decided to try harder. I had been given a valuable lesson
in *la bella figura*.

As August set in, the city emptied in anticipation of Ferragosto – the holiday that takes place on the fifteenth, which marks the feast of Assumption, and was also, from everything I had been told, simply the summer's most important event. Everything closed down as people fled to *il mare*. I found myself stranded, alone in the city. There was a silence to the days that washed up from the very streets to engulf the flat. People were away, windows were closed, the hum of traffic was dampened to almost nothing, there were no televisions blaring, no sounds and smells of meals being cooked, pans clattering on stoves, garlic fizzing and filling the air with the aroma of lunch. My neighbours were all away, even the old lady's windows were shuttered – she too was undoubtedly at the beach. The courtyard was quiet.

But the loneliness and depression that I dreaded coming with it didn't arrive. I somehow felt anchored by the emptiness of the city. While my Florence was deserted, the real Florence was boiling with people panting in the hot streets, sunburnt flesh spilling out of shorts and T-shirts. Even the market at Sant'Ambrogio had closed so I kept to my neighbourhood, circling ever closer to home, doing my thrice-weekly grocery shops at the little fruit and veg market in the Piazza Santo Spirito which lay beyond the Ponte Vecchio on my side of the river. I walked there early in the mornings to buy fresh white peaches and fat juicy mulberries before the sun got too hot. I snacked on the delicious fruit from Tuscan orchards: yellow and black plums oozing juice, blushing apricots, big dark cherries and several varieties of aromatic melon when I had the energy to carry one home.

I made salads designed to beat the heat, my favourite the fresh and aromatic panzanella which used that staple of Tuscan *cucina povera* – stale bread. I loved the act of making this dish and it kept well in the fridge, even more tasty the next day. I also spiced up my usual *tricolore* with dollops of cooked, cold farro – the ancient Italian grain which had fed the Roman army. Similar to spelt but more correctly called emmer, farro is a hulled wheat that predates spelt all the way back to early civilisation. My adventures in the kitchen were, perhaps, a small step for mankind but, for me, a quantum leap of culinary confidence.

Most places were shut but there were still some locals around – the local expats. Characters whose shadows had layered the days rose up out of the background to haunt San Niccolò in August, and I found myself shuffling down the street with Old Roberto, who was talking to me again now that Dino was forgotten. I discussed the day's headlines with a French artist who had a studio on the corner opposite the church. In the cool of the evening, he sat with his wife and baby outside the wine bar at that rose-tinted hour when we leftovers of San Niccolò drifted on to the street. Before long a mass of residents gathered, a mix of artists and layabouts. I met Tommaso, a painter who was once visited in a dream by Michelangelo's David and now painted nothing else. There was Donald, an ancient American who spent his days in his artist's studio outside the gate drinking, tottering over to us on unsteady legs in the gloaming. There was even a clown, Francesca from

Naples, who had fiery red hair and the loudest voice I had ever heard.

I joined this group in the evenings, drinking a glass of wine, the temperature finally bearable after the glaring heat of the day. Often a light breeze brushed past the tall saffron and mustard walls of the overhanging palazzi, bringing with it the scent of jasmine and sewers, the unique odour of Florence in deep summer.

As it grew cooler, I moved on from the bar and headed up into the hills for my evening walk. I had joined the rank of residents of San Niccolò, was a character glanced at by tourists in envy – the girl with the laptop outside Rifrullo, the one who got to live here, drink wine on the street. I liked this feeling of camaraderie, a silent bonding over our mutual obligation to whatever kept us here: poverty, work commitments, laziness. We spent our days hidden inside our flats, studios or workshops, avoiding the heat, our shutters closed against the insolent sun. With its dip in the sky, we headed out, and created our own living tableau on the street.

With Luigo's closed, Beppe gone and Cibreo shuttered up for the month, there were no daytime distractions and I was immersed in my writing, the deep quiet adding to my mood of quiet concentration. In the silent city, my world had reduced to the view from my window, and the Iranian revolution that was unfolding on the screen of my laptop.

My summertime reverie came to an abrupt end when an email crashed into my day. My past life had come back to get me. It was from a former colleague now working for a

rival publisher – no August by the sea for London's work-
ers – and she wrote brightly of a new magazine launch, of
all the market research and optimistic forecasts for its suc-
cess, of ABCs and profit projections. It was an ill-disguised
job offer. Would I, she wanted to know, be interested in
having a meeting to find out more?

Would I? I wondered. My first instinct was to protect
this creative space that I was in. But I could not avoid the
fact that I had not earnt a proper salary all year and would
at some point have to address my need for an income. I
wasn't ready to leave yet but it felt irresponsible to not
even look into potential job options. But at least I had
something to look forward to before I left.

I had a commission to review a hotel in the countryside
deep in the south of Tuscany, half an hour away from the
beach in the Maremma. After so much promise of *il mare*,
I decided that I would hire a car and take myself to the
beach on my way back to London.

A couple of hours of gliding along the motorway and I
was on the beach. It was windswept, scattered with drift-
wood, the air was soft with sea spray. At last I felt the sand
under my feet. I floated on the warm sea, thinking of all the
men who had promised to take me to *il mare* – that myth-
ical place in the Italian imagination – and how they had all
failed me. The peacock Beppe was not to be counted on,
the Pizza Boy had been too stingy, and the biggest liar of
all, Dino, I no longer cared enough about to speculate.

The Italian summer had not quite lived up to my expec-
tations, but here I was, on the shimmering Tuscan coast,
on a wild stretch of hidden beach with no umbrellas or

sun loungers in sight, and I was content to be alone. I felt entirely self-contained.

At the end of the afternoon, salty and relaxed, I drove through fields of sunflowers, their faces turned up to the sun, across the south of Tuscany to find the medieval castle-turned-hotel that I was to write about. Its stone ramparts rose up from a garden dotted with thick bushes of lavender and rosemary, terraces built into the hills, canopied by vines. Birdsong filled the air. A receptionist came out of the stone castle and greeted me, taking my bag and leading me to my suite across a courtyard scattered with metal tables and flower-embroidered canopies.

I was back in the world I had known so well, of high-octane luxury and opulence.

The grounds roamed over the dramatic slopes of the Maremman hillscape. There was an infinity pool perched on a cliff overlooking the valley, full of bursts of yellow Mediterranean broom with their attendant scent, and, after dropping my bags into a suite the same size as the whole of my flat in Florence, I jumped into the water for a sunset swim, watching the huge sky turn orange around me. I breathed it all in, the grand Tuscan sky, the humming valleys below, the scent of lavender, broom and jasmine on the breeze, wishing I could take it back to London with me.

A voice interrupted me. I turned round to see a short man in tweeds, his grey hair curling back from his forehead. He introduced himself as Carlo, the owner of the castle, and he invited me to join him and his wife for dinner on the terrace. An hour later, I peeled myself off the canopied four-poster bed where I lay sprawled and went into the courtyard which was now lit by flaming torches, a table set under an awning of vines where Carlo sat waiting. 'Ah,' he said as I approached. 'Come and try this.' He plucked a tiny grape from an overhanging bunch. 'Is called the *uva fragola* – the strawberry grape,' he offered it to me. I bit into the grape, which did indeed have a hint of strawberry, and as Carlo chatted, something about his manner niggled me. He reminded me of someone. Then his wife Aurelia appeared. Small and with bones as fine as a bird, Aurelia was every inch the elegant chatelaine in an understated linen suit, a steel-grey bob and generous smile. She was bearing a silver tray with three long flutes of champagne, greeting me warmly in excellent English. We sat down to eat, the table laden with produce from their garden, their vineyards, their herd of Chianina cows.

Throughout dinner, I was taken again by the way Carlo spoke, the things he said, his turns of phrase – so much about him seemed familiar. As the evening progressed, I racked my brain until it hit me: it was Dino. Other than physically, they were almost exactly the same. I was fascinated: the way Carlo delivered a line, his outlandish pronouncements, his humour, the toss of the head. As Aurelia talked, I was silently grappling with the possibility that so much of what I had found charming in Dino – the characteristics that I thought uniquely his – had been merely a Florentine archetype, and I had been too innocent to spot it. I was a foreigner here and, without understanding Florence and the language, I had been fair game.

Suddenly, Aurelia stopped mid-sentence, as if struck by inspiration – I could practically see the light bulb above her head. 'If you decide to come back to Florence,' she said, 'you must meet our friend Bernardo. He is a wonderful photographer – perhaps you can work together?' She scribbled his email address on a piece of paper and pressed it on me before running off to find some of his pictures. In her absence, Carlo, who had been regarding me wolfishly, leant over and said in a low growl, 'But just be friend with him, *ehn*? He has many kids and wives. Don't get involved, too many complications.'

I instantly pictured a roguish, handsome man who seduced models and carelessly impregnated every woman he saw. A flicker of interest sparked in a still-unreformed part of my mind, but I batted it away.

I stood on the edge of the pavement on Oxford Street. Buses rumbled by, and I stepped back to let them pass, dodging people jumping off, marching by. I looked around at all the buildings, the full flow of people going past, and took a breath full of exhaust fumes. I coughed. London felt claustrophobic, invasive, pressing in on me with its noises, skyscrapers and lack of horizons. It was way too fast, too furious. It made me breathless.

I stepped through the side streets of Soho and entered the grand lobby of the publishing house. People filed in and out, disappearing into the lifts; baby-faced young models sat awkwardly on the sofas waiting for castings. I gave my name to the receptionist and was pointed to the lifts. Upstairs I stepped out to be greeted by a sleek-haired

assistant with the vertiginous heels and Bambi walk that
marks out British fashionistas, who showed me into a
bright corner office. My ex-colleague greeted me warmly,
putting down a tall plastic cup with the remains of a murky
green juice, saying, 'My latest detox,' sucking the last of
it through a straw. 'It's all about kale now. It's pretty horrible,' pulling a face, the tip of her tongue working some
green bits out of her teeth. 'I've lost two pounds though,
and I am full of energy.' I could see make-up packed on sal-
low skin hiding dark circles under her eyes, teeth bleached
ultraviolet white. I had known her for years and the interview was straightforward: the publisher was launching
a new title and they wanted to know if I was interested
in being the editor. 'The launch editor,' my interviewer
trilled. 'And they are putting a minimum of five years into
it, so you have time to prove yourself.'

She broke off to remark with not entirely flattering
amazement on how much I had changed, how stylish, how
polished I looked. I was bemused. Finally she raised her
eyebrows expectantly: 'It's a chance to launch an important new brand. It's exciting. Are you up for it?'

A new magazine with the backing of one of the world's
slickest publishers, a whirl of activity and creativity.
I could feel it now: the adrenalin, the buzz of working
with some of the world's best-known photographers and
writers, being plugged into everything that was going on.
But it would be all-consuming too. There would be room
for nothing else. I looked out over the rooftops of Soho.
Five years, locked in, time to prove myself. A good salary,
a pension plan, paid holidays, performance incentives,

a spot in the company car park. I could come back in a blaze of glory – 'Everyone has been wondering where you've gone,' the interviewer confided in a low voice – resume my high-flying career, buy a flat somewhere leafy. I told her I would think about it and she shook my hand confidently, as if I was already on board. 'I'll think about it,' I said again. In the lift I found myself wondering who would be gathering on the street in San Niccolò for *aperitivo* tonight.

I had accepted some freelance work while in London. For a week I went back to something resembling my old life, my alarm clock next to my bed. I had not woken to an alarm all year, the bells of my tower were the closest thing I had. Now it was a shock but I took to setting my clock an hour earlier so I could stroll through the park for part of the way to work. The mornings were light and warm and the bus was quiet at that early hour. I got out in Regent's Park, walking along the canal and then past the zoo, passing giraffes with large pretty eyes in their pens next to the road, appreciating the time to myself. By the time I arrived at work – carrying my own flask of coffee which I made in my moka at home – I was perky and happy from my encounter with the giraffes and the walk along the beautiful flower-lined avenues in the park. I arrived on time and left on time, and always took an hour out for lunch no matter how much work was on my desk. I went to the little green opposite the office to eat my home-made lunch, and then went walking in Soho for the rest of the hour, looking up and around. I caught people's eye as they walked past, smiled, got a smile back. In the office, I went about my work without the overburden of responsibility and engaged with my colleagues, curious about who they were beyond these desks we were sharing. I met up with friends after work, sipping at cocktails on narrow streets under the late-summer sun, the evenings long and warm. I walked back home, meandering up through Regent's Park and past the pretty pastel-coloured houses of Primrose Hill.

What I had learnt in Italy about *bella figura* had come home to roost and I found unexpected beauty in London. Struggling with my suitcase up the stairs of the Tube station on my way home from the airport, I had been helped by an Englishman who carried my bag. It happened on my way back to the airport too. Such gallantry in London was as rare as a sunny day in February, and I was chuffed.

And yet I longed to be back on the streets of San Niccolò.

I sat on the bare floor of Kicca's flat, surrounded by boxes in the dying days of August. As we talked, I thought about Florence. It felt like home.

I looked at Kicca. 'I am going to stay,' I said. 'Maybe it's not the sensible thing to do, but honestly, it feels like the only sane thing to do. I am going to stay in Italy and see what happens.'

And then, contrary to the belief that had propelled me up the career ladder all those years, I said: 'I mean, it's only a job, right?' Kicca nodded sagely. 'There will be other jobs. It's not a whole life …'

Panzanella

Serves 2–4

1 **loaf day-old sourdough bread**
Red wine vinegar
1 **large white or red onion**
2 **large tomatoes, preferably beef heart, but any**
    sort will do. Judge by eye how much you need
    of different sorts
1 **cucumber**
Basil leaves
Best-quality extra-virgin olive oil
Sea salt and black pepper, to taste

Slice the sourdough bread: be careful here as the bread is
hard to cut and the knife can slip – my hands are scarred
from making panzanella! Place in a large oven dish and
pour on a mix of water and red wine vinegar – enough
to cover the bread and then some extra as it will all be
absorbed – you will need more than you think (1 tbsp vinegar to a cup of water).

Chop the onions into fine slices, put in a bowl and cover
with another mix of water and red wine vinegar. Leave for
a few hours, at least a couple.

When the bread has absorbed all the water, take each
slice, peel off the crusts and discard. Then squeeze out the
water, squashing the bread in your fists, and, massaging

it through your fingers, crumble it into a large bowl. Chop the tomatoes and add to the crumbled bread, along with any juice and seeds. Peel and chop the cucumber into small cubes and add. Drain the onion so there is no water remaining and add it to the bowl too. Tear up lots of basil leaves and add, then mix it all together.

Dress with a mix of olive oil and red wine vinegar, sprinkle on plenty of sea salt and a little bit of black pepper to taste, garnishing with some whole basil leaves.

Don't dress the panzanella so you can store it in the fridge – panzanella keeps well and the flavours deepen overnight. Leave in fridge for at least a couple of hours before serving – panzanella needs to be served well chilled.

Caprese 'farro' salad

Serves 2

150g farro
Sea salt, to taste
Best-quality extra-virgin olive oil
1 large buffalo mozzarella
**2 large tomatoes (if using smaller tomatoes,
    judge by eye how much you need)**
Large handful of basil leaves
Balsamic vinegar or lemon juice, to taste

Wash the farro in a bowl, passing plenty of water over it. Heat water in a large pan and salt when boiling. Add the farro and cook for around 30–40 minutes. Drain and let it cool, then mix with some olive oil so it doesn't stick together.

Slice the mozzarella, chop and add the tomatoes, and tear in some basil leaves. Dress with oil and either balsamic vinegar or lemon juice, season to taste, and serve.

9

SEPTEMBER
Stare in forma or how to never need a gym again

Produce in season: figs
Scent of the city: petrichor
Italian moment: watching a gig in Piazza Santa Croce
Italian word of the month: *alluvione*

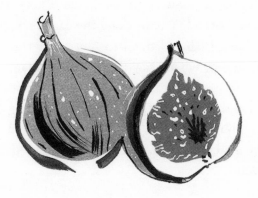

I came back to Florence in the first week of September. Summer was still in full swing but the deep heat and humidity had abated, the smell of drains was gone and there were fewer tour groups to dodge. The flat glare of August was replaced by a slanting light that gilded all the palazzos and towers. It was perfect, beautiful weather.

I was eager to be home, dragging my wheely suitcase behind me noisily from the train station. When I approached San Niccolò, Cristy appeared in her doorway to bow and scrape at me, Giuseppe the Gnarled Jeweller waved from the smoke-filled interior of his shop, Jack barked and the Rifrullo Pavarotti sang a snatch of '*il mio tesoro*' as I rounded the corner into my street. Monica tapped on the window from inside the bakery and I saw Guido give Gabriele a clip round the ear, sending him to take my bags. I handed them to him and let us into the building, smiling when I saw Giuseppe loping up.

I reached up on tiptoe and hugged Giuseppe. He was unshaven and his cheek tickled mine. Grinning broadly, he put me down. 'I heard the noise and thought – she is back!' he said, his arms spread wide. 'San Niccolò has missed you.'

I had a lot to catch up on. The changing of the month had been marked by the reopening of my favourite cafés, people reappearing at Rifrullo, looking relaxed, nut

brown, comparing tans, telling me stories of their holidays, their travels and adventures. In a rush of words,
Cristy told me that she had gone to visit friends in Salento,
Giuseppe the Gnarled Jeweller had returned home to
the marble mountains of Carrara with its own stretch of
Tuscan coast, Isidoro had been to his flat in Castiglione
della Pescaia on the Maremma coast and Beppe had gone
home to Puglia to visit his mother. Even the ever-skint
Luigo had managed a couple of weeks at a friend's house
in Viareggio. Propping up the bar at Cibreo, I looked at
the relaxed faces of the boys and understood the point of
the Italian summer and the August break. Everyone was
a better, nicer, browner version of themselves, as if they
had been dipped in honey.

I went to meet Antonella, excited to see her and *la
mamma*. Santa Croce was a mass of construction activity,
I had to dodge workmen as well as the usual throngs of
tourists in the piazza; it looked like a building site, complete with crane. There were rows of seats going up and a
stage being built in front of the basilica, much to Dante's
displeasure. Elaborate lighting rigs flanked the stage and
barriers were being erected to contain what was clearly
shaping up to be a makeshift open-air auditorium.

I stood under Antonella's window and looked up to see
her leaning out of the open window smoking and watching
the activity with a raised eyebrow. I asked what was going
on. '*Tesoro*, there is going to be a concert,' she announced.
'Every year they torture us with something. Last year it
was Roberto Benigni who ruined the summer murdering
the Divina Commedìa, *e mi aveva rotto i coglioni* ...' The

phrase translates as 'he broke my balls'. Antonella nodded.
'Yes,' she said, 'and I told him.'

'You told him?' I asked, remembering the lusty shouts
she had aimed at the players of the Calcio Storico from the
window.

'*Ma certo*,' she nodded. 'They can't expect to make this
casino under my window and not have to deal with me …'

I looked at her with admiration. Italian women had
the gift of righteous indignation. I was used to bending
into any shape necessary in order to accommodate other
people, no matter how much their behaviour annoyed
me – the curse of an Iranian upbringing. I looked at Anto
shrugging and spreading her hands and decided I still had
much to learn.

'Anyway, this year,' Antonella went on, 'it's George
Michael so at least we can dance. *Tesoro*, I am going to have
a party on the first night which is also your birthday, no?
So you must come …'

On my birthday, I clicked bravely over the bridge of graces to
Santa Croce in my sparkly heels, and worked my way through
the people scrambling to take their seats. Antonella buzzed
me in, greeted me with a glass of prosecco at her door and
guided me to her bedroom. She was wearing a sharp Helmut
Lang number – black, of course – accessorised with scarlet lipstick and yards of thick gold chains hanging from her
throat. There was a spread of perfectly toasted Tuscan crostini
on the dining-room table, in the centre of which sat the most
beautiful fig tart I had ever seen with a birthday candle in
its centre. 'Your birthday cake, *tesoro*,' said Anto, hugging me

as *la mamma* emerged from the kitchen with a tray of more crostini, putting them on the table before embracing me. The Adonises were out in force wearing particularly tight T-shirts, and they kissed me and hugged me to a chorus of *'auguri'*!

The crowd was roaring outside and we stepped through to the other room, taking our places at the windows as the lights flashed on the stage and spotlights roamed the audience. I had never seen Florence looking more beautiful – the evening sky was a dark blue velvet behind the facades of the palazzos illuminated with pink and blue lights, the dome of the Duomo peeked above the buildings and in all the windows around us there were people etched in the lights.

The orchestra struck up, lights twirled around the audience, and in a burst of dry ice, George Michael appeared, tiny against the looming facade of Santa Croce cathedral behind him. His voice filled the flat and we all started to dance and sing along to his songs. As the prosecco went down, the volume of Anto's comments – all aimed out of the window – went up. Finally, in the gap between two songs, Anto cupped her hands and shouted out: 'Oooooo Mi'hele' which had been her favourite catcall for a few songs now. The call landed in one of those moments of resounding silence, ricocheting around the square, bouncing off the walls. Audible laughter rippled through the crowd as hundreds of heads turned to look at us, and on the stage, even George Michael smiled. We heard a titter as he too turned towards our window, his dimple appearing in his cheek as his eyes met Antonella's and she blew him a kiss.

Figs were gloriously and stickily in season: on a roamingly long walk along the Lungarno, I stepped into a syrupy mess on the pavement, and cursing, I looked up to see a tree laden with figs boughing over me, threatening to bomb me with more ripe fruit. I reached up and plucked one, tore it in half and bit into its pink flesh, scraping it off the skin with my teeth. It was juicy and sweet as treacle. Later that afternoon, I came back with my straw basket and surreptitiously filled it with as many figs as I could reach.

Back in my kitchen I placed my figs carefully in the sink filled with water. They were mature and tender and I clearly had way too many – if I ate all these I ran the risk of spending the next few days chained to my loo. So I called Antonella to ask *la mamma* what I should do, and *la mamma* said, '*Ma figurati – devi fare la marmellata!*'

Yes, jam, of course. *La mamma* offered to help me and ten minutes later, I was in her kitchen sterilising jars in the oven while Antonella sat on the terrace – the only time of day that she would go out there was once the sun had dipped. Unlike most Italian women – whose *raison d'être* was to tan – Anto avoided direct sunlight as assiduously as a vampire; she had carried a small parasol at the height of the summer to protect her pale skin from the sun. 'You see,' she always said, 'no lines, *tesoro*. How many Italian women do you know my age who have cheeks as smooth as a – how you say it – baby's bottom?'

She was right. Aside from their sense of style, the thing that distinguished women of a certain age in this country was how crumpled their skin was from spending every weekend of the summer and all of August by the sea. Their dedication to sun worship, however, didn't mean Italians headed to parks – indeed, any sizeable sort of green space – as soon as there was a visible ray and strip off in their lunch breaks as we do in Britain. Apart from on the beach and by the pool, I had never seen Italians sunbathing. I asked Anto about this and she said, 'But my darling, because of the *bella figura*, of course. It's vulgar to take your clothes off in the middle of the city and bake your flesh in the sun.'

'But it's OK to literally fry yourself with oil at the beach?' On my one foray to the seaside I had seen teenage girls slathering each other generously in the stuff.

'Time and place, *tesoro*, time and place.'

I went into the kitchen where *la mamma* had the ingredients lined up: my figs were in a bowl of water in the sink, there was a bag of sugar and some lemons sliced in half. More surprisingly, there were also saucers containing, in turn, a pile of rosemary, cinnamon powder, some cardamom pods, a small knob of peeled ginger and a handful of cloves.

'All this?' I indicated, surprised. *La mamma* chuckled and let loose a torrent of broad Florentine of which I only understood 'figs' and 'variety'. I looked out pleadingly at Antonella nearby on the terrace. Without opening an eye, she told me that *la mamma* thought it would be fun to make two or three varieties and see which I liked the most: a plain one, a herb one and one with spices. *La mamma* handed me a knife, and ordered me to peel the skins of the figs. I watched as she set three pans on the hob and started to cook the fig flesh with sugar and the various other additions. My only other job was to stand over the pans and stir them while *la mamma* went and sat down in front of the TV and Antonella came to keep me company. Finally, it was time for *la mamma* to taste the three jams and declare them ready for their jars. I tried them all too: the plain one was gorgeously figgy, the herb version had a lovely tang of rosemary cutting the sweetness, while the one with the spices was layered with heat and piquancy. I loved them all and went home happily, eating pecorino cheese and the three different fig jams for supper that night.

One quiet Sunday afternoon, I accompanied Old Roberto to a shop on the via de Neri on the other side of the bridge. As we walked, the clouds that had been gathering overhead broke, one of those furious Florentine showers that made you doubt you would ever be dry again. We ducked into a shop selling pizza in little square slices, and I decided to eat some while we waited for the rain to stop.

But it didn't and, as we stood by the door, Old Roberto was silent, staring at the rain, visibly preoccupied. I asked if he was feeling all right and, stumbling, he told me that when it rained really hard like this, he started to have flashbacks to the flood of 1966 when the whole of Florence was submerged by water.

Old Roberto told me about the flood, how after days of rain the Arno had burst its banks and washed over the city in an oily surge of mud, carrying debris and even animals from the countryside into the streets and into people's homes, into the museums and piazzas. Roberto had been thirty years old, a man with a young family, living in the house that he still occupied on via San Niccolò, just one street back from the river.

We walked back over the Arno when the storm had passed. I regarded its fast-flowing waters with narrow eyes – it had always seemed so benign. I imagined the devastation the flood had caused, the most devastating natural disaster to befall the city. With her solid palazzos built like fortresses, Florence – solid, harmonious, ordered – seemed invulnerable, inviolable. And yet she was at the mercy of the Arno, so much of the world's most beautiful art sitting just yards from its banks.

I started to notice the plaques that charted the flood everywhere on palazzi, inside museums: *Il 4 Novembre 1966 l'acqua dell'Arno arrivo' qui*, they said. My walks became a mission to trace the flood and I thought of the massive clean-up job, the bravery of the people who had picked up brooms and mops and scrubbed that sticky oily mud off their city. The foreigners who had poured into the city to help restore the art, wash down the walls of the museums, donate clothes to those whose possessions had been destroyed. On one of my walks I visited the I Latini restaurant, the first to open after the flood, the family of the owner coming from the countryside near San Gimignano with olive oil, wine, whole sides of prosciutto and tonnes of bread, and how they had cleaned out their kitchen first so they could feed Florence. The anniversary was at the beginning of November, but these walks around town stitching together the monuments to the flood was my own little tribute to the city's most recent natural disaster. It was also my way of making sure that I never needed to visit a gym again.

Fig and ricotta tart

Makes 1 medium-sized tart

**Shortcrust pastry dough (I buy mine
   preprepared)**
450g fresh ricotta
3 eggs
¼ cup brown sugar (or local honey)
Orange zest
Cinnamon powder
8–10 fresh figs
Pistachios, to serve

Spread parchment paper on a baking sheet, then place
your shortcrust pastry dough on top and prick with a fork.
Preheat the oven to 200°C/375°F.

Make the filling by folding together the ricotta with two of
the eggs, the brown sugar or honey, some orange zest, and
a pinch of cinnamon powder.

Place the ricotta mixture on to the dough, spreading all
over except where you need to fold up the edges. Then
place the figs (cut in half and stalks removed) on top. Brush
the top with a beaten egg, then bake in the oven until
golden brown (20 minutes or so – check the bottom with
a spatula to make sure it has a nice brown colour). Let it
cool, then serve. You can also sprinkle a few pistachios on
top before serving.

Fig jam

Makes 2 large jars

1kg fresh figs
500g sugar
Juice and zest of 1 lemon
Sprig of rosemary or pinch of spices of
your choice (see page 219 for *la mamma*'s
suggestions)

Wash your figs, cut off the stalks, and carefully peel off the skin. In a large pan, combine with sugar and lemon juice, as well as a little lemon zest. Add whichever flavouring you choose – the herbs or spices – and bring to a simmering boil over a medium-low heat, stirring constantly.

Lower the heat and let the jam simmer, covered, for at least an hour, stirring occasionally. Remove the lid and continue simmering, stirring continuously until the mixture thickens.

Sterilise your jam jars and pour in the jam, removing the rosemary or spices. Since there is no pectin, this jam will keep for 3–4 weeks in the fridge before spoiling.

OCTOBER
Sprezzatura or the power of studied nonchalance

Produce in season: porcini mushrooms
Scent of the city: grapes
Italian moment: parking in the middle of the piazza
Italian word of the month: *Maremma maiala!*

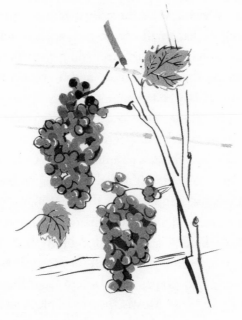

October was a month of light and shadow, the medieval walls imprinted with the silhouettes of cypress trees, the afternoon sun saturating the umbrella pines that lined the streets up to San Miniato. The temperature was that of a pleasant English summer but autumn's bounty filled the market. Antonio's stall overflowed with orange pumpkins, beige and dark green squashes in shapes I hadn't seen before. There were so many – from speckled marrows to bright yellow squashes shaped like stars – that even Antonio didn't know all their names.

Then there were the boxes of different mushrooms. There were porcini with their brown caps spread over broad, barky stalks, small cream prugnoli, which looked like champignons and were, according to Antonio, very popular during the Renaissance; and a colourful variety with smooth, glossy red-orange oval caps worn low over a golden stalk. These were ovoli, and, Antonio told me through a mime which I suspected was his favourite so far, they were also called Caesar's mushrooms for having been prized by the Romans. He filled up a paper bag with a handful of prugnoli and ovoli – the porcini were beyond my pocket – and told me to toss them lightly in a pan with a little oil, garlic and a herb called nipitella – calamint. Antonio instructed me to put it all on a bruschetta.

There were also grapes everywhere, signalling harvest time for the vineyards. Mostly they were black and red and very sweet and my favourite way to eat them became the *schiacciata con l'uva* when I was given some by Isidoro, a traditional schiacciata dotted with fat pieces of dark red grape.

I was eating one of these late one morning sitting outside Cibreo when my phone rang. I didn't recognise the number.

A gruff male voice, Italian. Heavily accented and audibly puffing on a cigarette. '*Ciao*, Kamin,' it said, 'I am Bernardo, friend of Carlo and Aurelia …'

The Complicated Bernardo! I had had an email from him while I was in London, a jumble of terrible English, telling me that he was away shooting but would like to meet when we were both back in Florence. I had shot off a quick reply with a date early in October and my phone number, and thought no more about it.

Bernardo, though, had obviously not forgotten. He was ringing me on the very date I had given him. He suggested meeting for lunch, telling me he was in the centre of Florence. I agreed and gulped down the last of the sweet schiacciata – I had just broken all the rules of Italian eating by having a pastry before lunch. It had taken obstinate insistence on my part to persuade Beppe to let me eat this so close to lunchtime, we had nearly had a row. The Italians believed so passionately in the good sense of their eating rules that they couldn't help but impress them on foreigners – namely me – at any given opportunity. For them, it was a public service, a humanitarian act. I had been educated well, and yet I was still capable of going dangerously rogue on the rules.

My misgivings on any more involvement with Italian men were overridden by the temptation of lunch somewhere new. Accepting a lunch invitation was always a good idea here.

'*Allora,* we meet at the Porcellino in half an hour?' he asked.

As I rounded the corner into the Mercato Nuovo, I hesitated when I caught sight of the man waiting in the appointed spot. He was nothing like the mental image of him I had; this Bernardo was shorter than I had imagined and broad-shouldered with a full head of curly brown hair, a generously lined face with a large Roman nose protruding over a clipped beard sprinkled with white. He was dressed in a light tweed jacket and jeans, muddy worker's boots on his feet; his fingers as he lifted the cigarette from his lips were covered in grazes and cuts. He was frowning slightly, deep in thought, preoccupied.

He hadn't seen me yet and for an instant I wondered if I should turn away and go home, but I pulled myself together and instead went up to him and said hello. He asked me if I too had rubbed the snout of the boar, as tourists were lined up to do in front of us. I shook my head. 'It brings luck,' explained Bernardo. 'If you are a visitor, you must do it.' We joined the line. The queue was slow-moving and conversation didn't flow. In fact, it was downright awkward. Bernardo groped painfully for every word in English; he seemed ill at ease. When it was finally our turn, he pulled out some coins which he tossed into the fountain of the boar while I gingerly touched the nose rubbed shiny by thousands of hands, my Virgo sensibilities challenged by placing my hand where so many germs must be lurking. 'So now,' he said, pointing to the coins, 'you will always come back to Florence.' And he gave me a smile so dazzling that it transformed his whole face.

Laying a hand on my elbow, he guided me round the corner to his car. He walked with a pronounced limp but nonetheless at such a fast pace that I had to trot to keep up. At the car he first went to the passenger door, which he opened for me before going round to his own side.

We drove through Florence, Bernardo explaining his limp, how an accident had left him with a leg so badly broken that he had spent several years in a wheelchair. 'You see,' he said, indicating a pink laminated square that was stuck to the window, 'I have this, is 'andicap pass. It means I can drive everywhere.' As if to prove the point, he turned sharply into the Piazza Santo Spirito, and, driving his car up into the middle of the square, he parked by the fountain. 'Are you sure this is OK?' I asked, looking dubiously at the chaotic parking, but Bernardo just walked on in his fast and lolloping pace.

The Piazza Santo Spirito was on my side of the river beyond the Ponte Vecchio. It was wide and leafy, overlooked by the church of Santo Spirito built by Brunelleschi. Its plain facade was unadorned, save for a perfect curlicue at the top. On the wide steps of the church was a ragtag of people: American teenagers drinking, Italian teenagers passing round joints, junkies with emaciated dogs, and tourists eating slices of pizza. Bars and restaurants were dotted around the square and the loggia of a hotel in a Renaissance palazzo stretched across one side. It was relaxed and bohemian and I loved Santo Spirito, often sitting on a stone bench under the shade of the acacia trees, watching the residents walk their dogs.

Bernardo led me through the square to a plain restaurant in the corner of the piazza. I peered at him over my menu. He had kept his scarf knotted around his neck, his head was held high as he looked down through his glasses at the menu, his big Roman nose dominating a face that reminded me of a portrait in the Uffizi. I rifled through the paintings in my head and, as he turned to the waiter and I caught his profile, it popped up. The Duke of Urbino, as painted by Piero della Francesca, in *Portraits of Federico da Montefeltro and His Wife Battista Sforza* hanging in the Uffizi. The hooded eyes, the hooked nose, the proud posture – here it was sitting across the table from me.

My own Duke of Urbino looked at me as the waiter returned. He ordered us a plate of fried porcini mushrooms, but otherwise he didn't help me with the menu. That was not the only difference with my meals with Dino. Instead of being solicitous, Bernardo was serious. Talking hesitantly in a sort of pseudo-English in which he anglicised Italian words, he told me about his photography, showing me the catalogue he had just been shooting for the Florentine fashion brand he worked for. He talked briefly of his three children, their two different mothers, the teenage son who lived with him, the two little girls who lived with another mother outside Florence. He also told me about his dogs, whose existence I had already guessed from the short white hairs on his jacket. Bernardo had, as well as the kids, some twenty dogs which he had bred – a lifelong passion from the age of fourteen. I nodded along politely, trying to decipher his English. Post-Dino, I was aware of how little I could contextualise a new person.

In London, every time I met someone new, there was an almost unconscious gathering of information that started the moment we shook hands – from the way they spoke, the vocabulary they used, the references they made. Here in Florence I had none of those references and it made me wary.

And yet his pictures were as good as the best that had crossed my desk; he had a particular way with light, a refined sensibility that reminded me of the luminous paintings I had seen in the Uffizi. I could see a real artist at work and I was intrigued. And so, uninspiring as our lunch was, when he suggested we go to the opera the following Friday, I accepted.

I love opera and I dressed up in a vintage Dior wool crêpe dress with a discreet neckline and classic full skirt that Antonella had pushed on me, declaring, 'Every girl needs a little black dress, *tesoro*, and no one did them better than Christian,' as if they had been personal friends. Opera was, of course, another Florentine invention: the oldest surviving opera was performed in Florence in 1600 at the Palazzo Pitti for the wedding of King Henry IV of France to Maria de' Medici. Bernardo's family owned one of two private boxes in the Teatro Comunale, and in honour of this illustrious occasion, I had taken down my sparkly strappy high-heeled sandals from the wall. I picked my way carefully across the street from my front door where Bernardo was waiting for me in his car. He leapt out and opened my door. I have always loved good manners. Brought up by Persian parents with strict adherence to a formal and

courteous culture, I have never lost the sense of dismay
every time one of my male friends slams the door in my
face in the name of equality.

Tonight Bernardo was more relaxed, the awkward manner gone. Approaching the theatre, we could find nowhere
to park, even with Bernardo's special pass. Eventually,
cursing, he said: 'Let me make a place,' and squeezed the
car into a half-space at an angle, mounting the pavement in
that inimitable Italian way.

I had been to the Teatro Comunale before, on one of my
first nights out with Dino as a couple. He had taken me
to a concert, we had sat in the stalls of the modern theatre surrounded by well-dressed people, my hand in his lap
under his coat caressing his thigh. I didn't remember much
more than that. Now Bernardo led me to the private box
which was at the end of a long corridor. He opened the
door with a small key and ushered me into a room with
a burgundy velvet sofa, two armchairs at the front of the
balcony, chairs dotted about. There was a wardrobe for our
coats. I handed Bernardo my jacket and sat down, watching
the scene below. The balcony was perched over the orchestra, on the side of the stage. It was a dramatically different vantage point, looking down into the orchestra pit and
back over the whole of the auditorium, watching people
take their seats in the stalls, along the circle, some glancing
up to look at me as I sat, floating above the stage.

Bernardo sat beside me in the other armchair, the music
rising up to envelop us, but as the first act went on, he
moved back to sit on the sofa. As Act One climaxed with
Rodolfo and Mimi's exquisite duet of '*O Soave Fanciulla*',

I was so thrilled by the purity of the voices ranging along the sweet romantic melody and the proximity of the singers, that I turned to Bernardo. He was sitting deep in the corner of the sofa, a blanket across his legs, fast asleep.

At the start of the interval, Bernardo woke up. 'When I was a child they brought us here once a week,' he told me. 'And I always fall asleep because,' moving cupped hands down by his thighs as if taking the weight of something very heavy, 'it was boring! Now is automatic – when I come here, I fall asleep. Every time!'

And sure enough, just like Pavlov's dog, as soon as we were back in the box and the music had started, he took a seat on the sofa again and within minutes was in a deep slumber.

'There was no pressure,' I explained to Luigo the next evening. 'It was actually really relaxing. The opera was absolutely beautiful and sitting up on top of the stage like that … And without having to worry about making some kind of impression, I enjoyed it much more! I mean this guy – I'm not sure if I like him, so actually, it was ideal!'

'Ah, *la sprezzatura!*' Luigo nodded wisely.

'Eh?' I blinked at him.

'*Allora, bella,*' he poured himself a beer, pushing a plate of *aperitivo* at me. 'Well, *la sprezzatura* is a sort of pretending not to care … what's that word?'

'Nonchalance?' I suggested.

'*Esatto, brava!*' He regarded me with approval. 'OK, so it was in a book published in fifteen-something. It was called something to do with courtier …' I chuckled. Luigo went on, 'OK, I don't remember all the details but you can go and ask your Internet. What's important is this idea that to be a perfect gentleman, you have to be, erm ...'

'Nonchalant?' I suggested again.

'*Brava!*' he said. 'So you see?' as if it was all very clear indeed.

'I need to know more,' I said, and he sighed.

'OK, so in the Renaissance, you know how rough the Tuscan aristocracy were?' I nodded. 'This guy wrote this book saying they should show restraint, that this was the way to go from being strangers to friends.' Seeing me frown he continued, 'So the handshake, for example, well, that's *sprezzatura* – it was a way for people to show themselves unarmed. The start of a cautious friendship.'

'So you are saying that he's being this thing – *sprezzatura*?' I asked.

'More than anything, I am saying that *la sprezzatura* is a good approach to a new friendship,' he said enigmatically. 'You might want to employ a little of it yourself.' And with that he went back behind the bar to serve a clutch of customers who had just walked in.

I investigated further. The author Luigo had referred to was Baldassare Castiglione, who had indeed written a book called *The Book of the Courtier* in 1528. *La sprezzatura* was a sort of code that advised restraint and gentleness in court behaviour – it laid the foundation of what has become accepted gentlemanly behaviour and attempted to regulate the wild ways of the Florentine aristocracy, who were far too apt to run each other through with swords.

Certainly this Bernardo seemed to be the very defin-
ition of *la sprezzatura*, showing no very overt signs of interest other than that he continued to ask me out. As his son,
Alessandro, lived with him, we mostly met during the day
when he was at school. A couple of weeks of mid-morning coffees and going to exhibitions gave me the chance
to practise *la sprezzatura,* keeping my restraint, the space
between us. It was easy to do, as I was not possessed by
the same wild attraction to him as I had been with Dino,
but slowly, calmly, every time we saw each other, I enjoyed
his company more, and he too became more relaxed and
more amusing each time and I began to see that under the
rough exterior lurked a gentleman.

Then one evening, after another concert at the Teatro
Comunale when he had, miraculously, not fallen asleep, I
found myself sitting in his car outside my building, locked
into one of those conversations that begins innocuously
and then somehow eats up the whole night. He managed to
turn the not-inconsiderable dramas of his life into a big joke
– his childhood in a castle in Chianti, the trials of his broken
leg, the failure of his marriages – painting their twists and
turns with light-hearted strokes, and I found myself laughing more than I had in ages. He didn't stop entertaining me
until the early hours when he left because he had to be up
in just a few hours to take Alessandro to school.

Every time I passed Dante I was reminded by the stone
book in his hand: by writing his great works he had made
the Tuscan dialect the official language of Italy. Until then

it had been a hotchpotch of dialects with Latin as the official language.

Florentine was certainly fruity, and Bernardo's language was colourful and peppered with Tuscan curses, many of which made no sense. The first time I heard him exclaim '*Maremma maiala*', I was perplexed. 'Pig from the Maremma?' I quizzed him and he nodded, laughing. Where Dino had taught me amorous phrases, Bernardo now taught me how to swear. *Maremma maiala* was followed up by *porca troia* (pig whore was the translation Bernardo offered for that one), *porca puttana* (from what I could make out, the same thing), *porca miseria* (pig misery). When I asked for a phrase that did not include pigs ('I am Muslim, you know,' I had joked), he taught me *che palle*. Meaning literally 'what balls', it was a wonderful catch-all curse that could be applied to almost anything, from something boring (accompanied by a teenage eye roll) to a real insult.

Bernardo was in my flat and my fridge was empty. Earlier that day he had taken me to a photography exhibition and, as I clicked my way around in my high-heeled boots, there was a flirty feeling between us. Dropping me home, he told me that Alessandro was out with his mother that night so he had a free evening. I invited him up to the flat. I was speaking with Kicca on Skype when he arrived and I kept the video call on so that she could meet him – I needed her opinion.

Bernardo, like Guido the Dramatic Idraulico, was astonished then delighted to see Kicca's disembodied head on my laptop on the kitchen table when he came in. Then, just like Guido, he sat down and started talking to her rapidly – the Italian default setting, the curiosity in people, the sociability, the volubility. Soon they were laughing and I searched the flat for something that would do for dinner.

When Bernardo saw me doing this he got up and headed to my fridge. '*Posso?*' he said and when I nodded, he opened it to find it virtually empty. I had not been to the market and I apologised.

'*Non ti preoccupare,*' he said, getting busy filling the pasta pan with water. Fifteen minutes later, we sat down, with Kicca still on the laptop, to a steaming dish of *pasta con aglio, olio e peperoncino* – pasta with garlic, oil and chilli, a Roman classic, Kicca told me, 'the best fast food there is!'

It was simple but also somehow creamy and tasty. I couldn't believe I hadn't come across such a handy dish before, made of the basics that existed in any Italian kitchen, even mine. I would add it to my repertoire. By the time I was making us coffee, Kicca had hung up and Bernardo and I were alone.

Suddenly I knew that Bernardo was going to kiss me. Having thought a few times over the past weeks that we were going to be just friends, tonight I was very aware of him as a full-blooded Italian male.

Yet, I wasn't sure about the wisdom of getting involved with someone with quite so much baggage, so I failed to cooperate. Every time I could have stood close, I ducked away. I busied myself round the flat and he followed me around like a confused puppy. Finally I decided to at least try out his kisses and joined him on the sofa.

And what kisses they were – long and lazy, deep and luxurious. I liked them and I kissed him for the rest of the evening, until it was time for him to go. Every time his hands moved on to my body, I steered him back to my lips, and he didn't insist. After hours of kissing – more than since being a teenager – my lips throbbed. So many kisses. Very fine kisses they were too – that much I knew. What I didn't know was how I felt about him yet.

I called Kicca back. 'I didn't think I'd hear from you tonight,' she said.

'Was it so obvious?' I asked.

She laughed. 'Well yes, there is such chemistry between you ...'

'There is?'

She laughed again. 'So what happened? I thought he would end up staying the night ...'

'Well, no, he can't because of his son. And, well, we kissed. But that's all.'

'How come?' Kicca seemed surprised.

'I wouldn't let it go any further,' I shrugged. 'I just don't know.'

'Darling,' she said, 'I think you are in denial. You told me he was not attractive and that you weren't attracted to him. But he's great, and really quite handsome, like a Renaissance painting! There was a real spark between you. I really liked him. He seems like a grown-up. You know what he said about his marriages?' I shook my head. 'He said – there comes a time when you have to put your balls on the table ...'

'What does that even mean?' I cried. The Italian obses-sion with balls had me mystified. It seemed like there was no situation in which a reference to their balls – even touching of – was inappropriate for an Italian man. Kicca laughed again.

'Well,' she scratched her head, 'I guess it means he has the guts to confront his mistakes. He said about his marriages that the first thing he had to do was accept his failure, to digest it and once again to put the balls on the table in order to go on …'

'OK,' I said. 'Well, you see! So he's got guts and I am risk averse. We're so different. He's all messy with his life and, well, you know me …'

'Neat in every way,' she laughed, 'a true Virgo.'

Kicca knew me and my perfectionist ways well. She knew that before setting off on a drive, I would carefully decant mineral water from a large bottle into a small one for the journey, she knew that I couldn't sleep at night if my bills weren't paid, that I had never been a day late with my rent and that no email was allowed to languish unanswered in my inbox for more than a day. She knew that my favourite domestic chore was washing up, for which I had to have a pair of rubber gloves to wear.

She knew all of this about me and she loved me anyway. So I could tell her anything.

'Kicca, I'm just not sure if this is what I want. I mean you know I am a cat—'

'A Persian cat,' she cut in.

'And he's a dog! I can't see how it could work. So that's why I just kissed him. And, my God, my lips are sore – I haven't kissed so much in decades …'

'Good kisser?' she asked.

I nodded. 'Actually, excellent, otherwise I would have thrown him out earlier ...'

'Darling,' she cut in, 'I know you're scared. After Dino, I am scared too – Dino didn't just happen to you, you know. But don't punish this guy cos of Dino. I don't think he's like that at all – I have a feeling he's genuine. And eventually you have to take a chance on someone new ...'

Two days later, on a particularly beautiful Saturday morning, I was in Bernardo's car, throwing caution to the wind. I had accepted his invitation for lunch at his house in the country and he had driven to Florence to pick me up. He hadn't told me much except that Alessandro was going to his mother's for the weekend and I hadn't asked how I would be able to get back.

We followed the river as it cut through a wide valley, the bank alongside us patchworked by allotments, the gardens whose produce filled the markets of Florence. Hills rose up around the valley, light illuminating fields, olive groves. We drove through the town of Pontassieve, named after a bridge built over the Arno in the sixteenth century, the place where the river Sieve flowed into the Arno. From here, Bernardo told me, we entered the valley of the river Sieve, a part of Tuscany that was still relatively unknown.

We followed the river to Rufina, a prosperous-looking place that, Bernardo said, grinning broadly, he loved for its lack of medieval walls, Renaissance fortresses, towers or historic churches. 'Here we have factories, not hilltop castles,' he laughed. Having grown up in the Pesa valley just south of Florence, with its splendid villas, turreted castles and refined, cultivated countryside – the picture-perfect Tuscan landscape that Dino had taken me to – Bernardo was in love with the lack of sophistication in this part of the province, its wildness, its wooded hills that rose up into the Apennines, its lack of pretension.

We drove out of Rufina and passed through another tiny hamlet. The air already felt different as we turned off onto a slip road with a sign for Monte Giovi – Jove's Mountain. The road passed under the arch of a railway bridge so small that I breathed in as we drove through, and then over the river Sieve along a short low bridge. Dragonflies darted on the surface of water so clear that the rocks on the riverbed were visible; the banks were wooded with beeches and oaks full of birdsong. As we crossed the bridge, the road narrowed, becoming steeper with twists and turns. I had the sense that we were leaving the ordinary world behind, entering an enchanted land of forests, soaring hills and mist-filled valleys. The road climbed, it was nothing like Chianti. It was big country – the sort of looming moun-tains that could be filled with wolves – squeezed dramat-ically into a small space, rucking up into steep hills and ridges over which fell dazzling beams of sunlight. The more we climbed, the more unreal it became, the road lined by chestnuts, pines, Mediterranean oaks and beeches, all backlit by the slanting sun.

After about five minutes, we had ascended high enough to see below the glistening river weaving through the jewel-green valley. Here we swung off the road into a vast sloping vineyard. We turned off the asphalted road on to a wide dirt track that cut through the vineyard into dense woods. Having climbed partway up Jove's Mountain, we were now traversing into the belly of one of its valleys. There was a vineyard on our left rising sharply uphill, and another on our right tumbling downhill. A group of red postboxes were placed by the entrance.

'Welcome to Colognole,' Bernardo said, his eyes dancing. 'This is the hunting reserve of the estate,' he pointed up the hill to our left where I could just make out the yellow walls of a large villa with a stone turreted tower perched above the vineyard. 'That's the big house, and here is woods full of animals, and the vineyards and olives, so you see.'

We drove slowly along the track and entered a dappled forest. There were bushes thick with undergrowth and wild flowers, a sloping coppice filled with large yellow sunflowers, facing the sun. Everything sparkled in the brilliant light.

Bernardo pulled down his window. 'You feel it,' he asked, sniffing loudly, 'how clean is the air?' — he pronounced it hair. 'Is no pollution 'ere, just mountain hair, *capito*?'

That must be why everything is so dazzling, I thought, squinting. I could see the Apennine mountains ranged purple on the horizon beyond the river, peaks laid over each other, soaring against the blue sky.

On a straight stretch of the track, with the hillside slanting up abruptly to our left and a vineyard dipping dramatically downhill to our right, Bernardo slowed down. 'There,' he said, pointing down the hill. 'That's my house.'

Sitting below us was a large stone house perched on top of a hill that rose up out of the river valley. Behind the house on the other side of the valley the hillside ascended, terraced in parts, thick with woods, the odd house nestling in the slope. Bernardo's house crowned the surrounding slopes, long and rectangular with grey stone walls, a roof of terracotta tiles. All along the front, I could make out fences and, in between them, running on little legs, small dogs rushing up and down. Suspended as the house seemed on this knoll, the dogs looked like they were floating in mid-air. Tall acacia trees boughed over the house, bright yellow leaves dancing in the breeze. It was quite a sight.

I turned to Bernardo. 'Wow,' I said. 'That's huge.'

'Nooo,' he laughed. 'That's not huge. You should see the Castello where I grew up. This is a simple country house. My first wife and I took it a long time ago, it was just a shell. We built everything – the kennels for the dogs, the runs outside, we made all that.' I examined his strong pro-file against this backdrop, the scarf wrapped around his neck, his head held high, thick curls backlit by the sun. He had never looked more relaxed to me, more settled in his skin.

He followed the track, taking a last sharp bend, crunch-ing over fallen leaves, down an even rougher and narrower track shaded by trees. There were thick woods on one side, Bernardo pointing to a clearing where a collection of beehives stood in a row. Boarded on the other side by the vineyard, the track led us to tall wooden gates, which Bernardo jumped out and opened, driving the car in, then getting out and closing them behind us. The car crunched up the gravel drive; there were large fenced runs on either side with dogs running up and down them and barking excitedly. Out of the front door of the house itself came a white dog, rushing up as we got out of the car. She reminded me of a small pig, walking as if on trotters, making snorting noises. At seeing Bernardo, she jumped up as if she had springs in her paws, turning around herself in tight little circles of elation, even bucking like a pony. She pointed her long muzzle up in the air and emitted a sound that could only be described as singing – a melodious sort of howl, a charming welcome-home song. And then she flung her muscular body at Bernardo who hugged her and kissed her long nose.

'This is Cocca,' he introduced us and the white dog came waddling over to me, wagging her tail. I patted her strong neck, caressed her soft muzzle. She was a miniature English bull terrier and she was Bernardo's dog.

'They are all my dogs, I breed them all,' he said, indicating the runs. 'But Cocca, she is my love. She lives in the house with us, she's part of the family.'

'Well, then,' I said, 'I hope she likes me.'

'Oh, Cocca is an angel,' he assured me as she poked my legs with her wet nose. 'She is sweet to everyone. That's why I called her Cocca – she's a *coccolona*.'

'What does that mean?' I asked.

'Oh, you will see!'

I looked at the white dog and Bernardo moving around the yard, and, with their funny walks and strong Roman noses, I giggled at the resemblance between dog and owner.

Colognole had a long yard with flowers in large terra-cotta pots placed around it. Outside the house, there was a collection of smaller runs, but across the yard, down a fenced-off slope which had stone stairs built into it, there was a large bank of grass with trees, leading down to a row of large, high-fenced dog runs, bordering the vineyard in front of the house. Behind the house, there were more spacious dog runs, and outside their fences, an orchard of chestnut trees and, beyond, the valley fell down to the river and the road that had brought us from Rufina.

It was delightful. The acacia trees provided shade, breezes rustling through their leaves. A long table and benches sat outside the house to the left of the front door; along the wall there were bright red geraniums, in sporadic flower.

'Come on, I show you upstairs.'

We entered into a grand hall, with a double-height ceiling beamed in the traditional Tuscan way. There was a large wooden door closed to the left, and another wooden door to the right that he pointed at, saying, 'This is the kennel, I show you later.'

In front of us was a stone staircase, which led up to a door painted red. Cocca was ahead of us, standing by the door, her right leg held up stiffly as she wagged her tail wildly, and when Bernardo opened the door, she raced in first. Before leading me upstairs, Bernardo paused just inside the door. 'Here,' he said, indicating the stone stairs by the door, 'is where I fell and broke my leg.' For a minute he was lost in the memory, muttering, 'You can't imagine the blood.'

I looked at the door painted red. He followed my
gaze. '*Eh si*,' he shrugged, 'maybe is a sort of symbol that
I painted the door red, no?'

Upstairs, what had looked like a large house from outside, was, in reality, a flat. At the top of the stairs, a spacious
hallway had several doors opening off it, but all, apart from
the one to the bathroom, were rooms in various states of
disrepair, filled with unwanted detritus of his past lives. A
corridor led off to the left through an arch, covered by very
thick, lined curtains. We stepped through these. The corridor went all the way to the end of the house. Immediately
on both the left and the right, wide brick-lined arches con-
nected the sitting room and kitchen. The sitting room on
the left had a high sloping brick ceiling, beamed with thick
pieces of wood. On the right a low wall sat between the
corridor and the kitchen, which was lined by wooden cupboards, the counter tops all the typical marble of an old-
fashioned Tuscan kitchen, pans and implements and mugs
hanging off hooks from a large wooden oven hood which
occupied the whole of one corner.

The sitting room was arranged round a huge fireplace,
with two dark red sofas and a low table, a television on a
corner table, a desk with Bernardo's computer along one
wall, in front of it a blue office chair. Cocca was already
up on the biggest sofa, burrowing into the large orange
striped cushions. Bernardo made a fire and I sat on the sofa
with Cocca, who instantly nuzzled into me, and started to
inch her way into my lap in such increments that before I
knew how, she was lying across my lap, pressing me down
with her not inconsiderable weight.

'Ah,' Bernardo laughed at me, 'so you see she is a *coccolona*.'

'A cuddle monster!' I exclaimed.

I watched Bernardo from the sofa, pinned under Cocca's weight, as he made us coffee. Here on his own territory, Bernardo was more confident, and much more sexy. And I was more susceptible to his kisses. So when he came over to the sofa and covered me in his long, lazy, luxurious kisses, and his hands roamed my body, I didn't stop him.

The next morning Bernardo slept. In sympathy with his gruelling weekly routine, getting up at five thirty every morning to get Alessandro to the train for school, I didn't try to wake him. I slid out of bed, slipped on his dressing gown and, in the kitchen, found a moka pot and the coffee. Cocca was fast asleep somewhere in one of the sofas, buried so completely under a pile of cushions that the only sign of her was loud snoring.

As the coffee percolated, I looked out at the vineyard and reflected on the day before. It had been full of surprises. There had been the delicious meals cooked by Bernardo: handmade *tagliatelle ai funghi porcini* for lunch, and a supper of *bistecca Fiorentina* cooked on the open fire and accompanied by a dish of peppers called *peperonata,* an exquisite mix of sweet and sour flavours followed by a salad of fresh wild leaves. There had been the Loo with a View, a small window in the bathroom which afforded the house's most sweeping views of the Apennine mountains, the river valley and terraced hills. There had been the cuddles with the affectionate and hilarious Cocca. And most of all, there had been Bernardo himself, who had swept me off to bed and kept me there all day.

The Complicated Bernardo had turned out to be a wonderful lover, tender and unhurried, luxuriating in the intimacy of the time we spent in bed. He had, in fact, been rather a revelation. A slow burner, he definitely improved on acquaintance, and when we weren't making love, we were laughing, sharing a slapstick humour that transcended our two languages.

The moka machine started to splutter. I heated up some milk and took my coffee outside. As I stepped out, a mass of sparrows rose in a flap of wings from the gravel. Their song filled the air, and there was the cooing of wood pigeons, the cluck of pheasants, a cock crowing somewhere. There were butterflies fluttering through the yard. The air was several degrees colder than in Florence, the freshness opening my lungs.

I sat on a bench by the long table and drank my coffee, taking it all in: the dogs, the sound of the breeze in the trees, the falling of the odd leaf, the layers of birdsong, the dazzling brightness of the sun, different greens all overlaid. I stood up and opened out my arms, taking a deep breath. I looked out over the vineyard and there, at the top, was a man, pointing a gun right at me.

I ducked, spilling my coffee, and rushed back inside. I ran up to the kitchen where Bernardo was filling a cup with coffee. I went to the window and peeked out – the man was still there. I pointed him out to Bernardo, and he shrugged lightly. 'Hunters,' he explained.

'But look, he's pointing right at us,' I cried.

'Is 'unting season, but don't worry, they haven't killed us yet.'

A shot went off, and the dogs started to bark wildly. All the peace was shattered. Bernardo opened the kitchen window, and, leaning on the ledge, he leant out.

'Ooooooooooo,' he called out in the loudest voice I have ever heard. The dogs immediately piped down, with just the odd straggler still yapping. 'Oooh, *allora?*' he demanded and there was silence – peace was restored. I chuckled to myself – the king dog, Bernardo, was the ruler of this canine kingdom.

We took our coffees back to bed and emerged from our bed-in only when it was time to go home. I kissed Cocca goodbye, she nuzzled me with her ears folded back against her head, raising a right paw, and laying it on my outstretched hand like a grand lady. I was delighted: 'I think we are friends,' I said.

We descended through the woods and down the hill in the last of the afternoon light. I pulled down the window, watching the magical wooded hills as we wound along the road. We were in a companionable silence, the atmosphere soft and dreamy.

As we followed the road down to the river, I let my eyes soak in all that green, the autumn colours just beginning, the red tinge to the vines. The fresh air was soft on my skin, the breeze caressed my cheek. We crossed the river, passed under the railway bridge and turned right on to the main road that took us back to Florence. I roused myself. Back to real life from the enchanted world of Bernardo.

Pasta con aglio, olio e peperoncino

Serves 2

4–5 cloves garlic
2–3 whole dried red chilli peppers (or red chilli flakes)
150–200g spaghetti
Best-quality extra-virgin olive oil
A small bunch of parsley, chopped
Sea salt and black pepper, to taste

Peel and chop the garlic roughly, chop off the chilli stalks, then cut them lengthways in half and slice (you can use red chilli flakes instead).

Fill a large pasta pan with water and bring to the boil, only then adding salt. Add the spaghetti and cook. Meanwhile, place the garlic and chilli pieces in a deep pan with the olive oil and cook on a medium-high heat till the garlic is translucent – 2–3 minutes only. Add the parsley and turn off the heat.

Just before the pasta is ready, when it is still a little chalky inside, drain, saving two cups of the pasta water, and add to the chilli and garlic mix, along with a cup of the reserved water. Place back on the heat, stirring constantly. Gradually add the other cup of water.

When the pasta finishes cooking with the garlic and chilli (3–4 minutes), season with salt and black pepper, and serve.

Tagliatelle ai funghi porcini

Serves 2

250g fresh porcini mushrooms
50g butter
1 clove garlic
Best-quality extra-virgin olive oil
150–200g fresh tagliatelle
Bunch of parsley or calamint

Carefully clean the mushrooms. Wipe the cap with a cloth, and scrape any earth out of the inside, chop off the woody bit at the bottom of the stalk. Try not to wash as they absorb water. If you have to do so, pass very quickly under cold water then dry immediately. Slice the mushrooms lengthways. Put the butter in a deep pan and melt on a low heat. Add the mushrooms and the garlic, peeled and smashed with the flat of a knife. Mix so each piece of mushroom is covered in butter. Then add a good glug of olive oil and allow to simmer on a low heat. Meanwhile take a large pasta pan and fill with water, bring to the boil, and add salt. Add the tagliatelle and just before it's ready (this will be quicker than dried pasta so don't overcook), add it to the mushrooms and stir together along with a cup of the pasta water, sprinkling with finely chopped parsley (or, better yet, calamint if you have it). Remove the garlic and serve immediately (you can put another cup of hot pasta water on the table to dribble on the dish if the tagliatelle is becoming dry).

Bistecca Fiorentina

Serves 1

1 T-bone steak
Best-quality extra-virgin olive oil
½ lemon
Sea salt and black pepper, to taste

The key is to use the best cut of T-bone steak you can find. Ideally, *bistecca* is cooked over an open fire, but you can also use a skillet pan. Heat the skillet on the hob until it is smoking, then add the steak, searing it on each side. The ideal *bistecca Fiorentina* is served very rare. Remove from the skillet, and serve, drizzling on some olive oil, lemon juice, and chunks of sea salt and black pepper.

Bernardo's peperonata

Serves 2–4

1kg green, yellow and red peppers (about 8–10 large peppers)
500ml vinegar (any basic vinegar is fine)
3–4 tbsp sugar, plus more to taste

Open and deseed the peppers carefully and remove the white edging on the ridges. Cut each pepper into four slices. Place in a large roasting pan, add the vinegar so the peppers are covered and there is a lot of liquid on top. Add sugar – the proportion is key so start with 3 or 4 tablespoons, then adjust to taste. You can cook the peppers in a medium-hot oven but Bernardo cooks them on the hob, usually over two rings at a medium-low heat which allows the liquid to simmer, stirring occasionally to make sure they don't burn. Be patient, you may need more than an hour, until the peppers have nearly caramelised. Then serve. This dish keeps very well, becoming more delicious overnight and is also good cold.

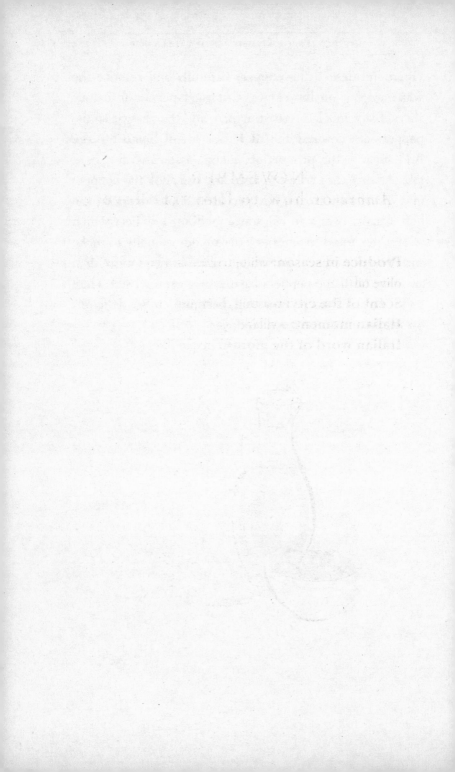

NOVEMBER
Amore or how to find true love

Produce in season: white truffles and green olive oil
Scent of the city: roasting chestnuts
Italian moment: a village *sagra*
Italian word of the month: *tranquillità*

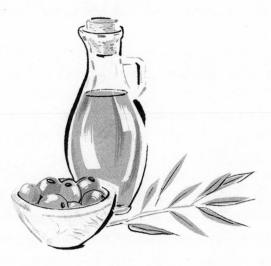

'Luigo, he actually licks his lips when he looks at me. I mean, every time, it's obviously totally unconscious. It's so sexy ...'

Luigo leant on the bar, listening to my babble. 'So, this is The One?'

I shook my head. 'Good God no!' I exclaimed. 'This is just fun! He's way too complicated to get involved with.' I was determined.

'OK.' Luigo was trying to look serious. 'But you have met his son, no?'

'Well, yes,' I admitted. 'Last weekend, before he took me home, we had to go and pick him up from his friend's house.'

I described to Luigo the drive through the Mugello, another spectacular part of Tuscany which Colognole bordered. 'The Medici came from there, you know,' I told him, proud of my new-found knowledge, 'and it's just gorgeous.'

'But how was his son?' Luigo asked, bringing me back to the point.

'Well, he was actually very sweet,' I said. We had arrived at a large country house and been shown into a kitchen with a big open fire, where we had sat drinking coffee with other parents as the kids came in. Bernardo's son was a slight boy, blond and blue-eyed, his colouring that of his Swedish mother. He had the same-shaped face as his father, a long nose, his hair curled around his forehead. He shook my hand and stood with his friends looking at me side-ways. The father of another boy started talking to me in English, a divorcee, he told me, also living in San Niccolò. He reached into his pocket and handed me a card with his phone number on it. 'Since we are neighbours,' he said, 'we should go for a drink some time.'

Bernardo moved closer to me then, slipping an arm around my waist. 'Luigo,' I said, 'the guy hit on me! Right there in front of Bernardo and all the kids! I didn't know what to say.'

'Are you still surprised by Italian men, *bella*?'

'They drove me back to Florence,' I told Luigo, 'and I invited them in for a cup of tea. His son seems quite grown up for a fifteen-year-old, but I guess that happens to kids of single parents, right?'

Luigo nodded sagely. 'So it went well?' he confirmed. 'The kid likes you, of course? I mean, you are from London and have an encyclopaedic knowledge of pop music ...'

It had gone well. We sat around my kitchen table drinking tea and talking. It was easy, sweet. And when Alessandro went to the loo, Bernardo regarded me with eyes so sentimental that, as soon as he opened his mouth, I deliberately talked over him, scared of what he would say. Alessandro came back into the room and the moment dissolved, but, despite my protestations that Bernardo was just for fun, I found myself so moved by the lone limping man and his shiny golden son, standing together on my threshold, that after shutting the door behind them I actually shed a tear.

They needed me, I had thought, but I didn't say this to Luigo. I hardly admitted it to myself, ignoring what my heart had told me so clearly that night: here, if you want it, is a family. Not perfect, not made by you, but anyway yours.

Did I want it? I pushed the question away and kept on seeing Bernardo for his fun value, for the epic bed-ins, and for the fact that he licked his lips every time he looked at me.

We were at a large supermarket on the way out of town. It was so long that I had been in one as big as this that I was wandering among the shelves like one hypnotised. The varieties of fruit and veg in the fresh section was mesmerising. I learnt to put on clear plastic gloves before touching anything, and how to weigh and price the produce. Bernardo's son had shown me all this, in between disappearing, only to jump out unexpectedly, Cato-like, at his father as he passed, setting off a mock martial-arts battle that moved through the aisles, dodging other shoppers, while I followed them, laughing.

Life in Colognole was quiet. Bernardo would cook, Alessandro helping, and all the while the ninja-style mock fights burst out. Before long I was involved too, side-kicking and karate-chopping as I laid the table. Then we had dinner, after which Alessandro would go to his room to do his homework and we would settle down in front of the fire with Cocca. Sometimes we roasted chestnuts, sometimes there was music – Bernardo playing me his favourite Italian songs – but often there was just quiet, into which the fire crackled and Cocca snored. The flames were compelling, Cocca had such a variety of strange and amusing noises, and Bernardo's embrace was so enveloping, that I was in danger of being permanently ruined by so much cosiness. The silence outside was deep, and I loved all those dogs sleeping downstairs; so much life, so much content- ment. It was profoundly tranquil, laced with nights lumi- nous with sensation and intimacy in Bernardo's bed.

Sometimes I stayed the next day too, doing nothing much apart from tumbling around in bed with Bernardo. From the window I watched the sun work its way down from its low post in the sky, before dipping below the top of the hill, illuminating the clouds, turning them a spec- trum of colours from vivid orange to a final delicate pink, the light of the gloaming infusing the whole yard a soft lilac. I hung out of the kitchen window to watch the pas- sages of light and colour, Bernardo holding on to my hips, saying: 'We don't want you to fall out, we just found you …'

Driving to Bernardo's home at night, the car lights picked out animals at the edge of the road: an owl perched on a fence; a porcupine waddling through the under- growth, its sharp quills fanned out; the long springy legs and white tail of a hare running away down the track; and once, a litter of baby wild boar with striped backs being led into the woods by the mother.

During the day, the vineyard was alive with the call of pheasants and their lazy flapping as they attempted lift-off, grouse littered the tracks, partridge tottered around and rabbits drove the dogs crazy by running up and down past their pens. Wood pigeons roosted in the rafters, kestrels and buzzards circled the skies and, on milder days, butter- flies fluttered across the garden. In the kitchen, there was honey from the beehives in the woods, and freshly pressed new 'green' olive oil from the trees of the estate. On my first vist Bernardo gave me a jar of honey and a bottle of green oil to take home. I was thrilled by both, knowing that the fine oil – bitter and fresh, an almost luminous green – came from the trees I could see around the house, and that the honey had been made from the flowers and trees outside.

Colognole was not just beautiful, it was pristine and uncontaminated, each lungful of air clean and sweet, the kind of place that in my former life I would have paid a lot of money to go to for a 'forest detox'. Add the crackling fire at night and the company of the funniest, strangest, sweetest dog, and it was a wrench to return to Florence.

But I made myself do so. I made myself say no as often as I could to Bernardo's offer to spend the night with him in Colognole – being a parent it was impossible for him to stay with me during the week. Alessandro seemed keen to have me come over too, we had gelled as a trio, but I was determined to keep the balance and not to lose my routine with the book. I knew from my experience with Dino how easy it would be. I kept this in mind even as my time with Bernardo began to feel more compelling. I stayed in touch with my reality, refused to lose my head and kept on the task of being an adult.

My flat, the kitchen, the fridge and everything in it stank of truffles. The weekend before we had attended a country *sagra* in the village of San Miniato, famous in Tuscany for its truffles. There had been dishes of tagliatelle served up on plastic plates at long tables laid in a marquee in the central square. It was packed and clamorous, the smell overpowering. Everyone, from granny to young child, had been tucking into the pasta, to which we had unlimited recourse for the ten euros we had paid on the door. I had been surprised by how little it cost to consume the world's most expensive food, and how few merchants were in the marquee selling their goods. I had assumed the *sagra* had been for the purposes of selling truffles, but I had been proved wrong. It was a true celebration, a chance for all the generations to enjoy at least one truffle-laced meal together, a truffle democracy.

I had come back from the *sagra* with a small lump, knotted and bumpy like a malignant growth, covered in dried mud, which I kept wrapped in kitchen paper in a glass jar. As instructed, I changed the paper twice a day, wiping the inside of the glass to catch any condensation: this was the key to keeping it fresh, that and not washing off the mud. I broke off a small bit by hand every day, brushed it clean with an old toothbrush, and then grated it with the special slicer we had bought, over a fried egg.

'The breakfast of kings,' declared Luigo when I told him, licking his lips at the mere mention of white truffles. I noticed that all my Italian friends had this subconscious reaction – even Giuseppe had come out of his studio, nose in the air, and knocked on my door, asking me if he was right in thinking he could smell truffles.

I apologised. 'It's such a tiny piece, but my God it stinks.' But he shook his head. 'No need to apologise,' he said. 'It's wonderful. You know that they say it is an aphrodisiac?' I nodded and asked him what he thought.

He pondered for a while. 'I'm not sure about the aphro-disiac part, but there is definitely some effect they have. Have you noticed?'

I had noticed. In the three days I had managed to make my little truffle last – having been warned that the longer it was kept the more it lost flavour – I had become aware of the involuntary salivating at the merest smell. I could feel the odour of the truffle travelling through my nostrils and into my sinuses, filling up my head, making me almost giddy. The man at the *sagra* had told me that when they were out hunting, they had to make sure the dogs didn't gobble down every truffle they found, and that tradition-ally the pigs that had been used to forage for them could locate them because they gave off the same scent that sows did when they were in season.

For days after I had finished the truffle, I could still smell it in my flat, and everything that had been in my fridge with the truffle tasted of truffle, as if the entire contents had been steeped in it – the butter, the cheese, even the milk. Even after everything was gone, there was a trace of it everywhere, as if it had permeated the inside of my nose.

Bernardo felt familiar. His warmth, his demonstrative nature, the way he took Alessandro's head in his hands and planted loud juicy kisses on the boy's cheek, no matter how much his son protested. He did the same to Cocca, who licked him back enthusiastically, her paws placed on his chest in a doggy embrace. It reminded me of my Iranian uncles, those loud, funny and sentimental men who couldn't let you walk past without grabbing you and covering you in kisses. And now here was Bernardo, who, as the mood took him, showed his love with the same loud smacking kisses.

I loved his lack of reserve. And yet, with me, he was not very demonstrative. When we were alone, I was in no doubt about his feelings but he had not yet included me in his public displays of affection, nor had he called me *amore*. After I told him about Dino, he had asked me if he had ever said that he loved me. I told him that while he hadn't said it explicitly, I felt it was implied, not least of all from the fact – and the way – that he called me *amore* all the time.

'This is very bad,' he said, frowning. '*Amore* is not a word to be used lightly. I only call people *amore* who I really love, *capito?*'

He was a man of his word. He called his son *amore*, he called Cocca *amore*, he even called some of the other dogs *amore* when he let them come up into the house for a bit of love and attention, but he had never called me *amore*. Not even in the heat of passion. I thought it a sign of my growing maturity that I was only slightly disappointed.

One Saturday morning, Bernardo took me to a village fifteen minutes the other way, going east. The road followed the river Sieve whose origins were in the higher reaches of the Tuscan-Emilian Apennines, and Dicomano was the gateway to the mountains. Situated at the crossroads of three of Tuscany's most beautiful and obscure areas – the Mugello, the Casentino and the Val di Sieve – Dicomano had me at the first turn of the road. A stone bridge forded the river, houses alongside the banks painted brick red and cadmium yellow, balconies hung with boxes of geraniums. The hills soared up, and the streets were abuzz with people. It was market day and we walked up into the centre of the village into a piazza packed with stalls. The road to the right of the piazza had an elegant long double loggia running on either side.

We walked around the stands, Bernardo buying fruit and vegetables, as adept at shopping as the fierce house-wives in Sant'Ambrogio market – life as a single parent meant he was an organised and thorough housekeeper. I found it wildly attractive. Every time I saw him clear up, get out the Hoover, wipe the table clean, fold his son's washing quite badly in a precarious pile, I went a little weak at the knees.

From the fruit and vegetable stall, he steered me across the square to a van with a counter in front of it piled high with little rounds of cheese. 'Pecorino,' he announced – the sheep's cheese that was so popular in Tuscany and which could be either quite fresh or very mature and hard. The two men behind the counter called out to Bernardo by name and they all stood around chatting. I couldn't under-stand all of it but I recognised enough words to realise that they were discussing politics and Berlusconi's recent rise to power. As they talked, the one called Carlo (I knew this because they were wearing aprons with their names embroidered into the top right corner) took out a roll of cheese and sliced into it, giving us both a small sliver to try: a pecorino with pieces of pear in it, one with tiny pieces of red chilli, another that had been aged for years, and, best of all, one with bits of truffle peppered through it. Each one was delicious. Beppe (the other cheese guy) held out a little mound of creamy white fresh ricotta cheese to me and I savoured it, nodding my appreciation.

When we got home, Bernardo put a little ricotta on a plate, drizzled on some of the honey from the hives outside and spooned some into my mouth. It was like manna from heaven and I closed my eyes with pleasure. Mountains, loggias and excellent cheese – Dicomano had it all.

Back in Florence, I was taking care of Cocca while Bernardo attended a meeting at the Kennel Club. I took her for a walk in the Piazza Demidoff in the chilly moon-lit night, intending to take her to meet Luigo. Cocca was pulling me inexorably towards the bridge, however, when Bernardo rang.

'*Com'e?*' he asked.

'Fine,' I said, 'except that she's trying to pull me over the bridge. She's so strong!'

'*Ah si,*' he said, chuckling. 'Well, she wants to go where there are people and show herself off. Be firm, don't worry about yanking her lead, see how much muscle' – he pronounced it 'muskle' – 'she has around her neck?'

He was right. Cocca had been a show dog, a world champion, as it happened, and as soon as we came to the city, she had an extra spring in her step, her gait super-perky. Bernardo had been breeding dogs since he was a teenager, it was something he had shared with his father, setting up their kennel then, and getting the accreditation from the Italian Kennel Club at the age of fifteen. At Colognole there was a room downstairs full of cups from all the shows he had won at over the past three decades. It was a passion that had shaped his life – he had met Alessandro's mother when he had visited her family kennel in Sweden and they had not just created Colognole's spacious kennel but also bred and showed generations of champions in the decade they were together.

I put the phone down on Bernardo and yanked at Cocca's lead. She reluctantly turned away from the bridge and followed me to Luigo's. I wanted to check in with him about my feelings for Bernardo, and I had brought him some *castagnaccio* from the bakery in Rufina, a sort of flat cake made of chestnut flour and sprinkled with pine nuts and rosemary which seemed to be everywhere now that it was the season for chestnuts.

'Well,' exclaimed Luigo as we walked in, coming round the front of the bar to pat Cocca, 'who's this?' and as Cocca jumped up to lick him, snorting and snuffing her pleasure, he laughed. 'Is it a pig or a dog?'

Cocca walked around everyone in the bar, sniffing at all their legs, wagging her tail and waving her paw like the Queen Mother on walkabout.

Luigo asked where Bernardo was.

'He's at the Kennel Club,' I said. He had just sent me a text in which he told me he would be back later than expected: there was 'much burocrazy' to deal with. I showed this to Luigo, laughing. 'Seems like an apt way to spell it, don't you think?' I loved Bernardo's rambunctious insistence on speaking English regardless of whether he knew the words or not. His texts were even more creative than his speech and they made me laugh, his multiple mistakes and malapropisms.

'Florentines,' I observed to Luigo, 'love their clubs. Bernardo has his Kennel Club. Dino had his tennis club—'

'And I have my gay clubs!' cut in Luigo.

I confided to Luigo that I was worried I was getting too involved with Bernardo too quickly. After all the men who never stayed long enough for me to actually unfold the double sofa bed, I told him, with Bernardo I had no opportunity to fold it up again. And not only did he stay the whole night when he could, but he brought his dog and his child with him too sometimes. He brought life – with all its mess and chaos – into mine.

'What are you scared of, *bella*?' Luigo asked.

'Well, earlier when he was driving away, I found myself trying to memorise his number plate ...'

Luigo leant on the bar encouragingly. 'So ...?' he said.

'Well, I was thinking – I should remember his number plate so that when he leaves me, I can identify his car ...'

For months I had squinted at every passing black Audi, wondering if Dino was inside.

Luigo walked over to my side of the bar and took my hands. 'You know, *bella*, Dino was a *stronzo*. I don't think this Bernardo is.'

'But how do I know, Luigo?' I pleaded with him. 'I'm getting so cosy with him. I mean, we sit on the sofa and hold hands and gaze into each other's eyes. His place is so lovely I never want to leave. This is all wrong!' My voice had risen to a pitch almost too high for human ears. Cocca was wagging her tail frantically.

'Don't panic!' Luigo stifled a smile. 'So you're comfortable with him! So you like him – maybe you even love him—'

I shook my head vigorously. 'No, Luigo! I don't. He's way too complicated – this is just fun! So, tell me, what can I do? I've kind of gotten here cos of *la sprezzatura* – what can I do to protect myself?'

Luigo chuckled. '*Bella*, there's nothing to do. Keep writing your book and keep being with your man. One does not have to exclude the other. So let go. Don't resist. Enjoy the man and his nice house and all those dogs and puppies.'

'But then what happens when I get attached to the house and the dogs and the kid? And then he leaves me and I am all alone …'

Luigo squeezed my hands. 'What if he doesn't leave you?' he said. 'Or what if you decide to leave him? It doesn't matter, *bella*. Have I taught you nothing about Italy and love? We love love and there is nothing shameful in loving and losing. Remember our relationships are "stories" – they are episodes, and however long or short, we give ourselves over fully to the story.'

I blinked at him.

'So you see, *bella*, it doesn't matter. If your story ends, you come and hang out with me until the next story starts. But,' he went on archly, 'I think what you are really scared of is not that it may end, but that it may not …'

Tagliolini with truffles

Serves 2

Sea salt, to taste
150–200g fresh tagliolini
4 tbsp butter

1 large white truffle, sliced super-fine
Fresh Parmesan, grated, to taste

Fill a large pasta pan with water and place on a high heat till boiling. Add salt and then fresh tagliolini. Just before the pasta is ready (remember fresh pasta cooks quickly), drain and reserve the water.

Melt the butter in a deep pan and add the tagliolini, along with a cup of the pasta water. Add the truffle and Parmesan and cook everything together for a minute, adding more pasta water if necessary. Remove from heat and serve immediately.

King's Breakfast: fried egg with white truffle

Serves 1

1 free-range egg
A knob of butter
½ small white truffle
Sea salt, to taste

Fry the egg in butter in a large pan until the white is crispy but the yolk is still runny. With a truffle cutter, slice some super-fine slices of white truffle on to the yolk, add some flakes of sea salt to taste, and serve.

1 2

DECEMBER
Stare insieme or how to be together

Produce in season: cavolo nero
Scent of the city: snow in the hills
Italian moment: Christmas in the Tuscan
countryside
Italian word of the month: *amore*

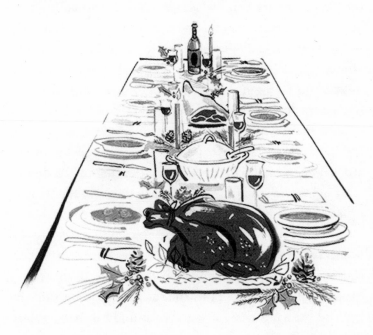

December arrived with enough of a chill in the air to justify the extravagant displays of winter dressing the Florentines had adopted since the start of November. Big puffy coats with hoods edged in fur, sheepskin-lined boots, gloves and thick-knit scarves encircled them so thoroughly that no hint of a cold wind could get in. Florentines were obsessed with catching chills – a mysterious concern even in the height of summer but the likelihood of which exponentially increased as the seasons turned colder. Old Roberto had been so concerned by my cavalier disregard for the possibility that he had given me a scarf all the way back in September when I had considered it still summer. In October, he had been shocked by my refusal to wear a winter coat. When I had coughed a couple of times, he had insisted on taking me to his doctor, whose surgery was a few doors down from Guido the Dramatic Idraulico.

Now that I was wearing my winter coat and the scarf he had given me, Old Roberto was finally satisfied with my attire, but that didn't stop him from urging me to tie the scarf tighter around my neck to make sure that the treacherous chill could not penetrate its folds.

There were frosts in the mornings, gilding the neighbourhood with a crisp layer of white. Occasional rain showers left bare branches embroidered with glistening droplets of water, backlit by the sun. Skeleton imprints of red and brown leaves were etched into the streets, ghosts of an autumn that was now conceding to winter.

There was a full programme of concerts and operas at the Teatro Comunale and we went often; I leant down over the balcony, rapt, while Bernardo dozed sporadically behind me. One night at the last minute Bernardo couldn't join me and he gave me the key to the family box. I invited Antonella and she came flanked by two of her tallest and most beautiful Adonises, extravagantly dressed in cloaks and stiff collars, one in a top hat, the other carrying an ornate walking stick and wearing a monocle.

As we settled into our seats, I told Antonella about Bernardo's emergency. 'One of his daughters is sick and her mother is freaking out, so he has gone to see if she needs to be taken to hospital,' I explained, reasonably. But I didn't feel that reasonable about it. Of course, I could not mind, the children came first. But his daughters and their mother were such shadowy figures in my life that every time their existence impacted me directly, I was not only surprised but a little put out.

As the orchestra took their seats beneath us, Antonella asked me how I liked his daughters.

'I haven't met them,' I said in a whisper – the conductor was holding up his baton. In answer to Anto's raised eyebrow I went on: 'They are little and he wants to protect them. That's fine by me, I am not sure I am ready to take on any more kids. And honestly, although he says everything is cool with their mother, I get the sense that it's not really.'

Whenever his second wife called, Bernardo went into another room to talk to her, lowering his voice, shutting the door. He had told me that on the weekends when she dropped them round to Colognole, she often stayed the whole day, stretching out her visit all the way to dinner.

I had wondered more than once if that meant she also stayed the night.

'Do you think there is still something between them?' hissed Anto as Tosca launched into an aria below us.

I had asked Bernardo this outright and he had assured me that he had no interest in her, had fallen out of love a long time ago. And when he called me on those weekends, very late at night or very early in the morning, his voice was intimate; he was clearly alone in his bed, and I had no reason to doubt him. 'No, but I get the impression that it's not as clean-cut as all that. I mean, he's told me that she – the mother – is very attached to the idea of having her family back together, but also that for him it's over.'

As Tosca's tragic fate unfolded, Antonella humming while the Adonises wept prettily, I told Anto of the Winds of Doubt which had recently started to blow through my time alone. They made me doubt my judgement, asked me if, after the experience with Dino, I could really trust Bernardo. They brought with them the chill of uncertainty, the whiff of confusion, the shiver of suspicion. They blew strongest on the weekends when he had his daughters, and I felt like the mistress, shut out of Colognole and hidden away in Florence, relegated in favour of the family.

Bernardo was open with his son about our relationship – at fifteen he considered him old enough, and anyway there wasn't much choice; he was a full-time single parent and daily parenting was very much his concern. From the start, I had understood that our involvement meant adopting – to some extent – also his son, and I had accepted this, and we got along well.

But then there was *le bimbe*, his two daughters, who lived with their mother in Chianti. They were young – just five and six – and their mum was a great mother, according to Bernardo. On the weekends that he had his daughters with him, he became unavailable apart from when they were asleep. He had told me just once that he didn't believe he should introduce them to new girlfriends unless he thought the relationship likely to last. 'I have made enough trouble for them, *capito?*' he had told me. 'I have hurt them enough …'

He had trailed off. Normally so open about his life, when it came to the end of his second marriage, Bernardo had told me only bare facts, and his face had closed in on itself. It was three years since he had left, but I felt instinctively that this was still a deep and private pain, and although inquisitive by nature, I didn't dig. It wasn't my business. It was his solitary and personal grief. I felt it, tucked away inside him, and I left it alone.

'I don't want to lie to them,' he had explained. 'I think they can tell, even if they don't understand … they are so young and at that age they imagine things, they make stories in their heads. I don't want to confuse them any more …'

I had got the message and, while it caused me some dis-comfort, I respected him for protecting his daughters, even if it was from himself. Especially if it was from himself.

And yet every other weekend, I struggled with my insecurity, with the fear that he would be seduced back into the family. And that's when the Winds of Doubt picked up and made me question everything.

On a drizzly Saturday morning, I discovered the Piazza Santissima Annunziata. The Ospedale degli Innocenti dominated one side of the piazza, Brunelleschi's loggia sheltering its front door. Above the columns, punctuating the arches, were della Robbia roundels of glazed terracotta, each one depicting a baby wrapped in swaddling, their arms spread by their sides as if lying down, glazed white on the vivid blue background, each baby in a different position, bearing a different expression. To the far left of the loggia there was a window with bars on it, surrounded by a fresco. Underneath it there was an inscription. 'For four centuries this was the wheel of the Innocents, secret refuge from misery and shame for those to whom charity never closed its door,' it said. This was where people left unwanted babies, those whose mothers had died in childbirth or were the results of the *droit du seigneur*. There was a slot that regulated the size of the child that could be left – this was how the baby entered the institution, left by a parent or midwife in a way that guaranteed the privacy of the act.

Built in the fifteenth century, the Ospedale had been a children's orphanage, started by a donation in 1419 from a 'merchant from Prato' and then managed by the Silk Guild of Florence who paid Brunelleschi to design one of the most beautifully proportioned examples of Renaissance architecture. The Innocenti was the first lay institution in the world to be dedicated entirely to infancy and childhood, centralising a service that had previously been scattered among hospices throughout Florence and the surrounding countryside. Children were taken in, documented, sent to wet nurses, educated and eventually integrated into the community through apprenticeships or domestic service. Indeed, there were still many Florentines bearing the surname Innocenti, testament to their forebears' starting life in this institution which even now provided children's social services to the city.

Children were very much on my mind. Bernardo was a father, a fact that I could not ignore. Christmas was in a few weeks and the complications of his arrangements as a twice-divorced father were making my head spin. Until now, his two families had proved quite useful to me; their existence dictated the time we spent together, provided the gaps and spaces I needed not to lose sight of my routine. I wrote for hours, visited the market, went for my walks, kept up with my friends, roamed around to find squares like this one. And so far this had worked well. I had managed to finish three chapters, which I had polished into a bundle with a proposal and consigned to my agent. Just yesterday she had written to me excitedly, telling me of interest from a couple of publishers.

'Come the new year,' she had written, 'I am sure this will turn into a deal. Isn't that a wonderful prospect for a new year?'

I had run to Luigo's with the news, he had popped open a prosecco and we had danced all night. Bernardo was already ensconced with *le bimbe* by then, so I had not yet told him. And now I was glad. I needed time to think. At the prospect of a book deal and staying on in Florence, my doubts grew.

I entered the cloisters first – one for men and one for women. They were inner courtyards framed by loggias, set with terracotta pots of lemon trees. They were arranged in the Islamic way, I noted, with the larger men's cloister set as soon as one entered the Ospedale while the women's cloister – long and narrow and tucked deep inside the belly of the building – was further in, protecting the women and children from the world as our old buildings in Iran did; the men's cloister placed to receive the outside world. The Renaissance architecture created by Filippo Brunelleschi reflected the one I was familiar with in Iran, adopting all the same themes with the vaulted arches, the loggias with their columns and inner and outer courtyards distinguished by gender.

I paused for a while in the shelter of the women's cloister. The soft rain fell silently into the long empty courtyard. I could imagine nurses crossing this cloister, bearing babies left in that doorway. In the museum of the Ospedale, I drank in the early Botticelli paintings glowing with gold, studied the *Adoration of the Magi*, Domenico Ghirlandaio's masterpiece, and a glorious blue and white Madonna and Child by Luca della Robbia. But what drew me was a glass case displaying a selection of mementos that had been left with the babies. These all dated from the first years of the Ospedale's opening, a fascinating array of the detritus of Renaissance life: little leather bookmarks, a cushioned fabric heart sewn with fat stitches, a broken coin – bits and pieces that the family could spare, objects of luck and also means of identity, something that would help the mother find her baby when she eventually came back to claim her child.

Those objects fascinated me, so telling of hope and heartbreak, shame and poverty, of the greatest sacrifice. A scrap of leather, a piece of broken medal, a heart made with fabric scraps – so insignificant in themselves but so precious to the mothers who, so many centuries ago, had laid these tarnished treasures next to the babies they had left for a better life, hoping that one day, through some miraculous change in circumstance, they could come back and claim their child, recognise it by the heart stitched together from rags and strung on a grubby ribbon round the neck. Transported back five centuries, I wept for these women, for the losses they had suffered, for the love contained in those scraps.

I wandered back out to the women's cloister and sat in the deep silence of that female space, letting my emotions settle. Questions that I normally avoided drifted up, questions about my own desires for a family, the ticking of the biological clock, whether I wanted to have a baby of my own. I could hear my mother's voice in my head: 'When are you going to settle down and have a family? You are already thirty-seven, soon it's going to be too late.'

My biological clock. I'd never heard mine. Or been aware of it ticking. Apparently we all have one, but where was mine? I had partied through my twenties, laughing out loud any time anyone asked me if I had kids. 'Me?' I would say with astonishment. I was taken aback that anyone should mistake me for an adult. Had my clock been ticking, I would never have heard it over the thumping bass anyway, from my place next to the loudest speaker.

In my thirties I had started to hear the clock. Not mine, but my friends'. Close girlfriends got pregnant, started families. The babies started arriving. They were magical, interesting, and they smelt good. I loved all our babies, and I collected quite a few godchildren. But I still didn't particularly yearn for one of my own.

One of my closest friends described her own wish for a baby as a tsunami of longing that had washed over her one day with such intensity that it had left her breathless. Another friend (the first of our group to have children) made me promise her that should I be approaching forty and still alone then she could help me choose a sperm donor and operate the turkey baster ... she seemed to think this was a perfectly normal offer but I was so appalled that I quietly cut her out of my life.

The only clock I heard was the one ticking out the remaining hours of one deadline after another. As my thirties had worn on, it seemed odd that there was no sign of this ticking, no tsunami, not even the faintest desire. No tick and definitely no tock. I had nothing against babies, and was a pretty good godmother to all my little ones. But, like any sane person, when they left after visiting my flat, I thanked God that I could give them back. I could find no emotion but relief in not having to live that chaotic life – one in which all one seemed to ever say was 'no' – and found the quiet of my home a comfort rather than an empty void, as the turkey-baster friend had called my child-free life.

And besides, there was no man – a crucial detail given that I had never contemplated having a baby without a partner. That, I knew with no doubt at all, was not for me.

And then, there was the longing to write. This was my tsunami of desire. Here I was, aged thirty-seven, and in the years that I should have been thinking urgently about finding a man and having a baby, I was preoccupying myself with giving birth to a book. Not just any book, but a book about my past and my family, my country Iran and the heartbreak, an opportunity to tell my family story and heal the wounds of the revolution and leaving Iran, life in exile.

So I sat in the women's cloister and tried to answer this question. Did I want a baby? Now that I had met a man I liked, was there anywhere in me a desire to make a family of my own?

And what about Bernardo? He had made it very clear from the beginning – no more marriages, no more kids. I respected his decision. Also, I didn't really think it was my problem. I had assumed that I would go back at the end of my year to something resembling my old life, albeit with better style.

But Bernardo was proving to be more charming than expected, kind, soft. I was unwilling to lose him just yet. And now that there was a potential deal for my book, I could perhaps justify this seductively slow and contented life in Florence.

All I wanted now was to go on with my writing, to go on excavating the historic pain of the revolution and exile, to bring it up to the golden Renaissance light and have it dissolve in this glorious beauty, where I had unwittingly

exiled myself. Apart from the sadness of not being able
to give my mother the grandchildren she so longed for, I
found absolutely no desire of my own.

I thought of Bernardo's scruffy country clothes and
scratched hands. He was the antithesis of Dino's mani-
cured elegance, and yet he was the authentic version of
what Dino had pretended to be – a real Florentine aristocrat, living in a big stone country house with lots of
dogs, vineyards outside the windows and wild boar in the
woods. His mother even lived in a castle and produced
her own olive oil and wine. Colognole was filled with life,
with love, with fecundity – all those kids, all those dogs,
constantly pregnant and giving birth, full of puppies. And
what of me? If I stayed, I would be the only female there
who would remain childless.

The rain had stopped. I walked through the square, my
head throbbing with these thoughts. I sat on a bench and
followed the gaze of the statue of Ferdinand I seated on his
horse to the legendary window that Giuseppe had told me
about. Situated on the second floor of the palazzo opposite the statue, there was a window which had remained
open ever since a lovelorn Renaissance bride had sat at it
to watch for the return of her husband from war. He never
came back, and she wasted away there. After her death, the
window resisted all attempts to be closed. Giuseppe had
also told me that if one followed the gaze of the mounted
Medici statue, it fell on the very same window, perhaps a
hint from the sculptor that the young lady had in fact been
the secret lover of Ferdinand I.

Florentine love stories, affairs and intrigues. I shook my head impatiently at the thoughts and marched home to immerse myself in my book instead.

In San Niccolò, I saw Giuseppe and, in answer to my casual enquiry of 'how are you?', he scratched his chin thoughtfully, pausing. 'I realised this morning,' said Giuseppe slowly, 'that I don't think I have ever occupied myself so fully …'

'Occupy myself fully,' I thought later as I sat on the corner sofa with my laptop. In London I had barely acknowledged myself, let alone known myself. The rush of appointments, overcommitted diary and intensity of stress had made me a stranger to myself, one who even refused to look at herself in the mirror. Now I got up and went to the bathroom, approaching the round mirror behind the basin with deliberate intent. I looked at myself. Curly black hair, glossy. Olive skin, smooth, plump. Light brown eyes, shiny. A curvaceous body that was trim and womanly. Most striking – the way I smiled at myself with the warmth reserved for a friend.

Here in Florence I had detoxed. I who had been so fond of spending money on faddish detoxes in London – none of which had shifted a kilo, erased a spot or brought a second's peace of mind – had come to carb-and-*gelato*-heavy Italy and undergone a true detoxification. One that had cleaned me out of the hyper-stimulation and stress which had depleted and drained my adrenal glands to the point that I had burnt out. By my learning to budget and live within my means, my redundancy money and small income from travel journalism had supported this gentle, unambitious life in Florence, which had, quietly and stealthily, calmed my body, and once my body was well again, my mind and my soul could heal. Instead of taking a pillbox full of vitamins and supplements, I now only took my daily dose of olive oil, and I had never felt better. And here I was, sitting on my sofa doing nothing at all but occupying myself fully.

I was in the flat, waiting for Bernardo. The table was laid with the prettiest crockery, spread upon a lovely clean tablecloth. A few sprigs of loquat blossom from Old Roberto's garden sat in a vase, filling the kitchen with their sweet scent. Ribollita was bubbling on the stove, a chicken was roasting in the oven. It was supposed to be our weekend together, but he had rung me the night before to say that he was taking *le bimbe* Christmas shopping today, and we had arranged for him to come to me afterwards for dinner.

The minutes ticked by, slowly turning into an hour. I called him, no answer. I started to fidget and turned off the oven. Another hour dragged by and I called him again. No answer. I spooned some ribollita into a bowl and forced down a few spoonfuls. A few more calls and messages and I put the whole roasted chicken into the fridge, furious. The months fell away and I was back in the turbulent, stifling days of the summer, a flashback to Dino and his perfidity, the way he would disappear for an evening then ring late in the night with an excuse, and then the way that he had suddenly vanished from my life. Bernardo was different, I had thought, but now, the Winds of Doubt whispered to me, he was no more reliable than Dino, probably in bed with his ex, as he had been for the past months, enjoying stringing me along while rebuilding his relationship with her, putting his family back together.

I threw on my coat and marched to Luigo's. I found him getting out Christmas decorations for the bar and offered to help. As we were stringing the lights, he asked me whether I was spending Christmas with Bernardo.

'It's looking very cosy with him, *bella*,' he said, winking at me. 'And now you have a family of your own, will you spend the holidays together?' He loved to tease me about acquiring 'a second-hand child'.

'No, Luigo,' I said, bursting into hot tears. 'That's all over. I've decided.'

Luigo led me to a table and sat me down with a glass of water. 'What happened, *bella*?' He was puzzled. 'It was going so well.'

I told him, and as he started to say, 'He's scared ...' I cut him off.

'No no, this isn't happening again. This time, I am going to decide. Bernardo and his menagerie can take a running jump. I'm done ...'

And I was so determined that, when Bernardo rang me first thing on Sunday morning, I switched off the phone and rolled over in bed. This time, I would be the one who was unreachable.

I ignored his calls and messages all day until, coming home in the early evening from a walk, I found him waiting for me at my door. 'Thank God you are OK,' he said with visible relief. 'I was worried. I wanted to apologise for last night ...'

I led him silently up the stairs to my flat. As we sat down in the kitchen, I wanted to throw the cold chicken at him, but I said nothing and sat down waiting for him to explain, watching him closely as he told me that he had fallen asleep on the sofa.

'You know how that happens,' he said, and indeed I did. Quite often on a Saturday evening, he would doze off on the sofa in front of the fire, worn out from the week. I asked about *le bimbe*, about their mum, about his day with them.

'*Le bimbe*, they stayed the night with me,' he said, his face open, guileless. 'It was easier because their mother had a date last night ... we had an early dinner and I sat down to send you a message and then, I woke up this morning. The phone had run out of battery.'

'So their mother had a date?' I asked.

He grinned. 'Well, it seems that since I told her about you, she has decided to move on too.'

'Wait,' I held up my hand, surprised. 'You told her about me?'

'Well, yes,' he shrugged. 'I told her last week. Eventually, I want you to meet *le bimbe*, so it's right to prepare her, give her some time to get used to that, *capito*?'

With a gust, the Winds of Doubt – which now sounded like my mother's voice – hit me between the eyes with the reality of Bernardo's life. He may not have been cheating on me last night, but he had collapsed, exhausted. These two months of fun were, inexorably, bringing me towards the truth. Overburdened, tired, at the beck and call of a small army of other people who would always come first, who would always come before me.

'Forgive me, *cara*,' he said sincerely. 'It's been a long time since I had someone. I don't really like casual relationships. I hope you feel like I do.' He blinked and I held my breath. 'I wanted anyway to come and invite you to spend Christmas with us. What do you say?'

'What did you say?' cried Luigo, unable to bear the suspence any longer.

I drew a deep breath. 'I said, I need some time to think. I'll call you in a week or two when I have made up my mind.'

'When you have decided about Christmas, you mean?' Luigo quizzed me.

'When I have decided about him, I mean,' I told him, as Luigo gasped with the unexpected drama of it all.

Luigo was not the only one to be surprised. I had surprised myself. And Bernardo had looked like I had slapped him in the face.

I hadn't tried to explain and he hadn't pushed me to. He had left and I had gone to bed early, falling into an agitated sleep.

The day after, I woke up expecting that sinking feeling you get when a relationship has ended. Instead, I felt calm and perfectly collected. I set about breakfast, squeezing red oranges, sipping tea and buttering toast, gazing out over the tower, when the phone rang.

'Have you moved into the castle yet?' Christobel chirped. I sat down with my tea and poured out my concerns. She listened carefully, apart from a whoop that broke out of her when I told her about the publishers interested in my book.

'I don't understand what the problem is,' she said eventually. 'You can stay in the flat as long as you want and carry on writing your book and see how things go with Bernardo. No?'

'But Christobel, all his baggage. I don't know ...'

'Listen, darling,' she said, 'the fact is, everyone has baggage. Anyone you are going to meet at this age is going to have baggage. It's just that some people's baggage you can see – like Bernardo – and some, you can't – like Dino. But it's there all the same.'

I nodded silently. She went on as if she could see me: 'Take it from me, no one is perfect. And OK, so Bernardo has all these ex-wives and kids, but he sounds like a good man.' I nodded again, murmuring my assent. 'And these past couple of months you have been so happy. Not in that giddy way like with the dastardly Dino, but in a real way. Think about it, take your time, but remember, good men like him are rare, and at least he admits his mistakes. Make sure you aren't throwing something good away just because you are scared that it might turn into a real relationship ...'

I sat alone in my flat, finding it very empty. All that life in my space – the huge presence of Bernardo, the muscular body of Cocca weighing on my legs as we slept at night, her myriad snorts and noises, the radiating warmth of his body, the blond boy in the other bedroom. I sat on the sofa next to the twinkling lights I had strung up around the room and distractedly picked at the pinzimonio I had made. Even Giuseppe was away. I clung to my routines, preparing multi-course meals that absorbed my thoughts and time, plugging away at the book and walking all over the city. As each step fell on the cobbles trodden by so many lovers over the centuries, I thought: 'Nearly a year has passed. What will I do? What's my life and what's my future?'

I thought about my past, what I had left in London. Before leaving I had cut out all the articles I had written over the years for various magazines and filed them neatly in chronological order inside plastic pockets. Two files covering a fifteen-year period, all my writing laid out. I flicked through them now. What did they amount to? Was this all I had to show for my life so far?

Because there had been nothing else. No relationship. No children. No house and a mortgage. Plenty of other things, like friends and family, little godchildren and the whole of London waiting to divert me. But nothing intimate, warm. Nothing really outside of my career ambitions. Just, as I remembered it, a lot of being alone. Loneliness – I had never called it that. But now looking back I could see that it had crushed me. That sense of emptiness, of being tired of doing everything alone.

Here in Florence I had been solitary but not crushingly lonely. I had found a liberating lack of ambition that had emphasised the ordinary and everyday. It had given me the space to create, that reassuring absence of judgement in Florence, the fact that what you did was not what defined you. It had allowed me to stop doing and discover how to just be. London was much too stimulating for the state of undistracted calm I needed to create something as long and complicated as a book. Although it felt counter-intuitive, the slow pace of life in Florence had sharpened my senses, not dulled them.

And since Bernardo's appearance, life had become infinitely richer. All that life – the puppies, the dogs, the boy who needed me as much as his father did, the other children that perhaps one day I would meet too. My mother's voice piped up inside my head: this is not your family, you should make your own, and this man will never give you that ... No, he would never give me that, he had said as much. But, foolish or not, perhaps this was not a problem. Marriage was too distant a possibility, and children of my own – well, I was facing up to the fact that the model of womanhood presented to me by my mother was not the one I wished for. I didn't want to be defined by my relationship and my children – for my body to be the territory of others, to be my identity. It came to me in a flash – I want to be free. Free of that kind of belonging that children bring. I hardly knew what this meant, but I felt it instinctively – the desire to make my own life, at any age and any stage of my existence, to be creative in ways other than through procreation. And I also felt instinctively that Bernardo would give me that freedom.

At the end of the agreed two weeks, I sat quite alone on a bench along the *viale* from Piazzale Michelangelo, the church of San Miniato behind me, and let my eyes drift over the city, once so new and uncharted, now familiar, always awe-inspiring.

I recalled the first time that I had seen this view, standing with the other tourists at sunset up at Piazzale: the city bound by its medieval walls, outside it the hills and valleys scattered with grand villas inset with delicate loggias, cypress trees on the horizon, the emerald grass dotted with silver-green olive trees like pom-poms. There were mists weaving through this valley that bordered the ancient walls punctuated with turrets, and on the other side, the terracotta roofs of Florence packed together, its churches, the bell tower of San Niccolò, the orange walls of the Palazzo Serristori behind my flat. The silver line of the river cut through the buildings, threading through the arches of the different bridges. On the other side there was the watchtower of the Palazzo Vecchio, the brick bell tower of Santa Croce. And squatting like a giant in the middle of it all was the white mass of the cathedral, its vast red dome, the marble tower with its bells. Around it all the wooded hills dotted with villas and lights.

I was no longer ticking off monuments. Woven into the view were my memories of my year, the homes of my friends, the sites of my adventures. Scenes of my year in Florence rose up like ghosts: meeting Antonella outside the gay bar behind Santa Croce, Beppe kissing me on the doorstep of Cibreo, singing with Francesca at the checkout of Pegna, miming my shopping needs to Antonio in the market. I saw myself walking arm in arm with Dino through the gate of Porta Romana, thrilling with the anticipation of his kiss, and I watched the preoccupied-looking Bernardo gazing at me as I reached out to gingerly touch the snout of the Porcellino.

Looking to the hills of the Casentino as they were etched, hazy and delicate, on the eastern horizon of the Arno, I smiled. Somewhere there, I thought, is a man (and a shiny blond boy and a funny white dog) who wants me and to whom I feel like I could belong.

I meditated on Bernardo's patience in waiting for my decision, his bravery with his heart – this heart that had been battered and broken, bruised and knocked about so many times, so often and by so many people. And yet, here he was again, with his heart in his hands, cracked and imperfect as it was. He was not waiting for a distant day when it would be whole and perfect. He was offering it to me as it was, with no pretence at papering over its cracks, but with honesty and transparency – be that for another month or a lifetime, he was not holding any bit of it in reserve.

At first I had found him thoughtless, careless with himself. Then, as the days passed and my steps echoed on untold cobbles, I realised that he was brave. It wasn't that he didn't feel fear. He let his fear and panic co-exist but not overtake his heart, his desire to be with me. Unlike Nader, his reaction was not to run back to safer arms. Unlike Dino, he didn't create a fantasy that he controlled and then – the ultimate demonstration of his dominance – leave without a word. Unlike Beppe, he was a man with understanding of life. Bernardo was, perhaps, the first grown-up man I had been involved with.

And his bravery inspired me to be brave too. To take a risk, not knowing how it would work out, what might come in the future. Once more, I decided to step off the edge of

the cliff. A cliff with a Renaissance façade but a cliff nonetheless. But this time, I was not stepping off the cliff alone.
This time, I had someone by my side, holding my hand,
taking that step with me. It made the move no less dangerous but it did make it infinitely more companionable.

The only choice, I realised, was to stay.

My phone rang. It was Bernardo. We had not talked in
two weeks, and my days had paled. I had come to see his
complications not so much as annoyances, but as riches
that embroidered my life, gilding my quiet daily routine
with an abundance of characters and energies.

I answered with a smile in my voice, and Bernardo
smiled back down the phone – I could hear it. He told
me that he was at Rifrullo, asking where I was. 'Wait ten
minutes,' I urged, 'I will be right there, I'm just up by San
Miniato.'

I walked happily to the winding road that led back down
to San Niccolò, practically skipping in my excitement to
tell Bernardo that I would spend Christmas with them.
As for the rest, I decided I had better confirm things with
Christobel before telling him, just to be sure.

As I was rounding a bend, I stopped to let a car go past,
a smile on my lips as I thought of Bernardo. I looked at
the car as it drew closer and slowed down to take the
sharp bend – it was a black Audi, the window was wound
down on the driver's side, and there, so close that I could
have reached out and touched him, was Dino. He was
staring so fixedly ahead that I knew he had seen me, and
as he passed, I laughed out loud. All those months of
peering into the windows of every Audi, thinking of all

the things I would say, even if it meant shouting into his window. And now, just when I could not have cared less about him, when I was skipping joyfully around thinking of Bernardo, finally he had appeared, to bear witness to my happiness. It couldn't have been more perfect if I had dreamt it up myself.

It was the night before Christmas Eve and Florence was decked out in her festive finery. She was prettier than ever. Cascades of lights hung over the streets of the *centro*, and the *giglio* of Florence, made of pinpoints of light, was suspended between the buildings. The Piazza della Repubblica displayed an enormous Christmas tree hung with red *gigli*, and another twinkled in front of the Duomo, Christmas songs emitting from deep within it. A wooden manger to one side of the cathedral bore exquisitely sculpted terracotta figures of the holy family placed among bales of straw. My side of the river competed with the centre, with an enormous Christmas tree festooned with lights overlooking the city from Piazzale Michelangelo and the tower of San Niccolò was lit up in reds and blues. A group of carol singers from the English church spent evenings traversing the Oltrarno carrying a fake gas lamp and singing English carols, and a festival of lights illuminated monuments around the city every night.

We drove to Colognole that night, through the dark country road skirting the river, passing Rufina with its own show of Christmas lights and displays of winter flowers lining the streets. We followed the road as it led us over the river and twisted up the mountain – Bernardo's mountain

– and, rounding a bend, he slammed on the brakes as a herd of deer broke out of the bushes. They passed immediately in front of the car, and, as we held our breath, one turned and looked right at us. 'Good God,' I said, 'is Santa coming up behind them?'

'You see, Kamin,' he said, grinning and placing a hand on my knee, 'the city is beautiful, but Colognole is magic.'

He had picked up a real tree and wreath for the front door. They were sitting in the front entrance of the house. 'I can't believe you haven't done any decorations yet,' I turned to Bernardo.

He shook his head, telling me he wasn't a fan of Christmas. 'Yes, but Alessandro?' I cried. He assured me that his son too didn't care but I refused to believe it. 'I bet he'll love doing all this,' I promised. 'Just wait ...'

The next morning Alessandro willingly agreed to help me decorate the house. He led me through all the rooms that were shut up, full of boxes and a disorder of things, and we unearthed the Christmas decorations. We went for a walk into the woods to find holly and ivy. And as we gathered up armfuls of spiky leaves, Alessandro said shyly: 'I'm glad you are here for Christmas. My father has invited other friends and it will be fun this year.' I looked at the boy, shiny as a newly minted gold coin in the woods, and my heart went out to him. I patted his back. 'Yes, we will have fun,' I said.

We spent the rest of the afternoon weaving the foliage into corners as Bernardo set the table for the next day, explaining to me that Christmas Eve was the *vigilia di Natale*, it was customary to see in midnight together. 'When I was little they took us to church,' he said, 'but now for us is enough to be together until it passes into Christmas. We can have supper in front of the fire.'

Joining us on Christmas Day were his best friend and his family. 'You will like Gaetano,' he told me, 'he was educated in England, he speaks really good English.'

A son of an impoverished Sicilian noble family, Gaetano was, according to Bernardo, a true gentleman, 'but you could never tell from his clothes. He is even more rough than me, *cara*,' he said. When they met, Gaetano had been living with his parents, helping out with his father's business but deeply unhappy. Bernardo had encouraged him to leave the job and follow his heart.

'And what did his heart want?' I asked.

'Gaetano is the best falconer I have seen,' he said. 'He has a way with birds that's like ...'

'You with the dogs?' I interjected.

'Actually, much better. But be ready. Gaetano loves his birds, he takes them everywhere and his pockets are full of rats' tails ... And he has Cocca's son. He's called Cocco, you will meet him, he's got a black patch over one eye.'

Our *vigilia* was spent in front of the fire, Bernardo cooking us steaks on the flames while Alessandro and I finished up the decorating, finally tying a red bow around Cocca's thick neck. After supper, Bernardo fetched a Monopoly board and the three of us played a raucous game together until, at just gone midnight, we all retired to bed, wishing each other a Merry Christmas. Hours later, I slipped quietly out of bed and placed the presents I had brought with me under the tree, hanging up three stockings above the fireplace. I sneaked back to bed, feeling pleased with the execution of my role as Father Christmas.

The morning came, wrapped in mist. I made us all breakfast, and when Bernardo and Alessandro got up, I pointed to the fireplace. 'Father Christmas must have come in the night,' I said to them, and I watched as the boy excitedly took down the stockings.

'You see,' I said to Bernardo as he watched the boy empty his stocking with all the eagerness of a young child, 'he does like Christmas after all.' Bernardo slipped an arm around me and pulled me close. 'Thank you,' he said, looking into my eyes, 'you are a sweet woman.' And I melted into him.

Bernardo was busy in the kitchen from first thing, making a traditional Italian Christmas lunch. He first placed the *cappone* (cockerel) into a large pan with plenty of water and *odori* – a mix of carrots, celery, onions and parsley – to boil. Calling out instructions to Alessandro over his shoulder, the two of them whirled around the kitchen together, preparing the leg of ham and placing the turkey he had picked up from the butcher into the oven. Alessandro peeled potatoes and I cleaned the vegetables: Brussels sprouts, carrots and bunches of cavolo nero. There was also pork to roast and tortellini to cook in the broth made from the water of the boiled *cappone*. When he deemed this ready, after hours on the stove, I held the sieve while Bernardo poured in the water, throwing away the remains as he transferred the broth to another pan. Once this was done, all we had to do was wait for his guests, who, he assured me, would be late. I retired to get dressed and, when I reappeared, I found Bernardo and Alessandro eyeing up the presents under the tree.

'What's this?' he demanded. 'I thought I said no presents?'

'It's Christmas!' I hadn't been able to help myself. 'There have to be presents ...' I loved rituals and celebrations, couldn't let Christmas pass without some parcels to be opened, convinced that, whatever he said, his son was still enough of a child to be thrilled by Christmas presents.

'In that case ...' Bernardo said and disappeared into the bedroom, coming back with a small box which he placed into my hands. 'Happy Christmas, *cara*,' he said, kissing me on the cheek. I tore open the paper excitedly, and opened the box to find a pair of exquisite earrings, cylinders of delicately wrought silver wrapped around balls of turquoise, my favourite stone. I clapped my hands in delight. 'They're gorgeous,' I hugged him, 'how did you know?'

Bernardo smiled and indicated Alessandro. 'Well, he helped me!' and Alessandro came and hugged me too, grinning from ear to ear. I put them on, to their admiring cries. I was still flushed with pleasure when I saw Cocca out of the corner of my eye, walking in along the corridor. But there was something over her eye and I was about to go and examine it when I saw Cocca coming out of the kitchen the opposite way, at the same time. I was about to rub my own eyes: there were two white dogs now, nose to nose, like a mirror reflection except that the new one had a black patch over his eye.

'Cocco!' exclaimed Bernardo. '*Dai*, they are here,' he said and, with that, a tall man with a soft fleshy face and thinning wispy brown hair walked in, holding a baby. His wife was right behind him, tall and slim with short hair, leading a toddler by the hand. In the commotion of introductions and hugs and greetings that followed, Cocca executed a bull-terrier dance in the middle of the kitchen. Sniffing at her son, she reared up on her hind legs, spinning around and bucking mid-turn as Cocco copied her, then she snorted in excitement before raising her muzzle and letting out a long song of joy, rushing from one person to another, poking our legs with her nose as her tail wagged furiously.

Gaetano shook my hand, looking at me with piercing blue eyes, a smile across his broad face. 'I have heard a lot about you,' he said in a perfect English accent. Instantly likeable, Gaetano was everything Bernardo had described. A big, cosy man, he was warm and funny and his wife Ilenia was, he told me as he introduced us, his falconer assistant.

'Ah yes,' she said in heavily accented English, taking the baby from his arms, 'before we had these ones,' indicating the kids, 'we were parents to twenty hunting birds.' She turned and pointed to a big cage that had been placed at the end of the corridor.

'You see,' she said, rolling her eyes, 'he brought his new baby with him ...' and Gaetano went to the cage and slowly opened the door, placing a gauntlet on his hand, coaxing out a large bird which sank its claws into the leather as it climbed out on to his arm.

I gasped. As Gaetano got up, holding his arm aloft, the enormous bird perched on it spread its wings. They spanned the whole width of the corridor.

'Royal eagle,' said Gaetano. 'We had to bring him, we only got him a couple of weeks ago and I didn't want to leave him alone. Want a demonstration?'

'Oh, yes please!' I said, looking at the proud creature as he perched, his head turning this way and that, his yellow eyes impassive.

'*Dai*,' said Bernardo. 'You go and fly the bird and I will put on the tortellini ...'

I followed Gaetano outside. Ilenia stayed with the baby to help Bernardo but the children came too. Gaetano placed the eagle on a post and positioned himself in the widest part of the yard. Telling us to stand back, he took something out of one pocket which he then tied on a string. I peered at this, realising that it was a dead mouse.

I leant in towards Bernardo's son. 'So he really does have pockets full of dead mice?' I asked, wincing, and the boy laughed. 'Oh yes,' he said, 'that's nothing. Wait till you see the other bits ...'

'Even on Christmas Day?' I was as amused as I was fascinated and disgusted.

The boy laughed. 'That's Gaetano ...'

Gaetano released the bird which spread its enormous wings, soaring into the sky, above the trees, over the vineyard. The mist of early morning had lifted, leaving a bright but bitterly cold day. The eagle swooped through the sky, turning and rushing back towards us, where Gaetano was swinging the rope with the dead mouse, and the eagle dived down, chasing the bait, passing low over our heads. I felt the wind on my face from its giant wings, heard the feathers fluttering, saw the majesty of the eagle's flight close up. Gaetano made it pass us a few more times before bringing him in, the big bird landing silently on Gaetano's upheld arm. Holding it aloft, Gaetano instructed Bernardo's son to bring him something from upstairs and, when the boy reappeared with another leather gauntlet, Gaetano asked me if I wanted to hold the bird.

'Is it safe?' I asked. The eagle was huge, bigger than Gaetano's toddler, and I instinctively shied away from it, from those cold eyes and sharp, curling beak. But Gaetano assured me that it was OK, and as I donned the glove, he came close and handed me the fine chain that he had clipped on to one of its claws.

'Hold this loose, and I will hand him over,' he instructed me, and as I did what he said, the bird, in a flap of his giant wings, skipped from Gaetano's wrist to mine.

I held up my arm, looking at the eagle. It didn't move, but turned its head, and looked right at me. Our eyes locked, and I saw the eagle's flicker – he was looking me up and down. I was mesmerised, I had never been so close to something so wild. I had the feeling he was sizing me up, much in the same way that Antonella checked me out whenever she saw me. An Italian bird, I thought, as Gaetano took the eagle back from my arm. I felt elated by this incredible encounter.

When we arrived back upstairs, the places were set and the food was steaming on the table. A soup tureen was full of *tortellini al brodo*, the turkey sat in the middle

surrounded by roast potatoes with rosemary, the vegetables were placed all around it, and at the other end of the
table, there was another large dish with the roast pork
sitting on it. There were two boxes of panettone on the
sideboard. Bernardo had made a centrepiece from the
poinsettia and holly I had brought, and there were tall red
candles burning on either side in silver candleholders I
hadn't seen before. An exquisite crystal carafe filled with
red wine sat on the side and in the other room a fire was
crackling in the chimney. It was beautiful.

'I've never seen so much food,' I said as we took our
seats, 'I thought we were over-the-top in England!'

'We are in Italy,' laughed Bernardo. 'We like our food,
you know ...'

We all sat at the table, the baby in a high chair next
to Ilenia, Cocca and Cocco at our feet, the eagle perched
on the low wall by the kitchen, watching. Occasionally
Gaetano got up and, reaching deep into his pockets,
brought out a mouse's foot or a tail and fed it to the bird.
I sat back and watched the scene, and I smiled. So this, I
thought, is a regular Christmas with Bernardo.

On New Year's Eve, Bernardo was once more at my door,
licking his lips as he looked at me in my red Fontana Sisters
dress and sparkly heels. '*Ma quanto sei bella*,' he said, his
eyes devouring me, and I flushed with pleasure – he was
usually so taciturn – for an Italian man – that when he
made these compliments, they meant so much more.

I had accepted Antonella's invitation for dinner and,
although I was fluttering to feel his skin on mine and we

were both tempted to see in the New Year in an epic bed-in, we jumped into the car and headed over the bridge. Florence was all lit up, full of people, the atmosphere crackling with laughter.

Bernardo had just taken his daughters back home and dropped Alessandro off with friends. He had been there since Boxing Day with all his children. He looked content, the lines on his face softened by the days with his family.

'I look round the table last night,' he told me, 'and I think, *mamma mia*, all these people are made by me!' He glowed with happiness and I felt a stab of jealousy. Not at the love that he had for his children but at not being part of the scene. As if reading my mind, he went on: 'Only person missing was you, *cara* …' and the feeling melted away. There was no stinginess to Bernardo, I thought, no need to fight others for portions of him. He was generous with his love; his heart just stretched to encompass more people to care for.

The Piazza Santa Croce was once more cordoned off. This time there was no stage, but a station for fireworks in the middle of the square, complete with sandbags all around and a couple of fire engines at the ready. Once more from Antonella's window I would have ringside seats for one of Florence's best shows – its New Year's fireworks display, this year to be launched from the middle of her piazza.

Anto flung open the door, champagne glass and cigarette in hand. She too was wearing red – the first time I had seen her in a colour – and her hair had been freshly, sharply cut. She hugged me and, on being introduced to

Bernardo, embraced him too, ushering us in. The flat was full of people; there was a full turn-out of Adonises, mostly crowded round *la mamma* who was sitting, resplendent in sequins, on a chair by the buffet table spread with food. I could see Luigo in the crowd and there, in a corner, was Giuseppe.

'*Amore*, come in,' Anto was at my elbow, 'and eat some lentils,' indicating the dishes placed at either end of the table. 'It is traditional ...'

'Means you will have money all year,' cut in Bernardo.

'I'd better have several plates then!' I said.

I went around the room hugging all my friends. Luigo whispered in my ear, 'So, *bella*, what's new?' and I told him about the latest conversation with Christobel, the decision I had made.

'So ...?' Luigo arched a brow, glancing at Bernardo, who was laughing uproariously with *la mamma* across the room.

'Shhhh,' I put a finger on his lips. 'I haven't told him yet.' Antonella joined us, and Luigo told her the news. '*Amore!*' she exclaimed, hugging me. '*Brava!* You've chosen well.' She indicated Bernardo. 'I like him. But you better watch out, *la mamma* seems to love him,' as another peal of laughter burst out of *la mamma* and Bernardo. Then, turning to Luigo, she said: '*Allora, ti pago dopo* ...'

'Wait,' I cried. 'Pay him? Did you guys have a bet?'

'*Cazzo*,' cursed Anto, 'your Italian has improved and we don't have a secret language any more ...' She gave me another hug. 'OK, yes, but is only a joke. I say you are too scared, but Luigo here,' she clapped a hand on his shoulder while Luigo pouted, 'he is a true romantic.'

'That's because, *bella*, I have seen you together,' said Luigo, sipping his drink. 'Now, *basta*, let's go dance!'

Antonella's bedroom had been transformed into a dance floor. Her few pieces of furniture had been removed, the bed tucked into the corner of the room and piled with cushions. 'Is chill-out area,' said Anto, indicating the pile of silk on which lounged two gorgeous Adonises. In the hallway between the sitting room and the bedroom, there was a deck and a DJ, an Adonis twiddling the controls while arranging his earphones around his hair, and disco lights flashed in the bedroom.

'This is amazing,' I said to Anto as she pushed me on to the 'dance floor'. And we danced, Adonises appearing to twirl us around. I whirled through the evening, at different points dancing with Luigo, Antonella; even Giuseppe came and waved his long limbs around in a gloriously arrhythmic way. Bernardo accompanied *la mamma* into the room, swaying her in his arms, telling me over his shoulder as he circled her past: 'I am in love with this woman ...'

As midnight approached, we gathered by the windows, putting the lights out. At the stroke of midnight the Duomo's church bells rang, echoing through the city, ricocheting off the walls around the piazza as Antonella's guests burst to life, whooping and jumping up and down, everyone hugging each other. Holding on to Bernardo, I kissed him as the firework display whizzed into life, the lights exploding in the night sky, illuminating the city, the dome, the facade of the church. We leant out of the window together to watch the sparks overhead.

'Happy New Year, Bernardo,' I stroked his beard. 'What are your intentions for the new year?'

He gave me an intense look. '*Di stare insieme* ...' he said. 'My intention is to stay with you ...' He stopped and swallowed hard. My heart skipped, his vulnerability disarmed me. It was time to tell him about the potential book deal and my new arrangement with Christobel. Leaning in closer, I told him that I had decided to stay in Florence to keep on writing my book. 'At least until it's done. And then we will see ...'

His face wreathed into the biggest smile, he pulled me close. We kissed as fireworks lit up our faces and then he looked deep into my eyes again and said:

'Happy New Year, *amore.*'

And then:

'*Amore mio* ...'

Tortellini with capon broth

Serves 4

2 onions
2 cloves garlic
3 sticks celery
2 carrots
Best-quality extra-virgin olive oil
1 capon
Sea salt and black pepper, to taste
300g fresh tortellini

For the broth, make a soffritto, gently frying the finely chopped onions, garlic, celery and carrots in olive oil in a deep pan. Once the soffritto is cooked and aromatic, fill the pan with water and add the capon. Season with sea salt and black pepper and let it simmer for a couple of hours or more, spooning off any fat or scum that forms at the top.

Remove the capon from the pan – you can serve the delicious white flavourful meat separately but never in the broth – and sieve the water to get rid of the vegetables so you are left with a clear broth. Transfer the broth to another deep pan, throw in the tortellini (we buy ours from a specialist fresh-pasta maker but if you want to make your own, I recommend Marcella Hazan's recipe) and bring to the boil. It doesn't need long so watch out not to overcook – just a few minutes.

Serve the broth and enjoy – this is the Italian version of chicken soup, *mamma*'s traditional cure-all!

Cavolo nero with oil and lemon

Serves 2

2 bunches cavolo nero (other types of kale can be used)
Sea salt and black pepper, to taste
Best-quality extra-virgin olive oil
Juice of ½ lemon
1 clove chopped garlic (optional)

Wash thoroughly and dry your cavolo nero. Remove the fattest part of the stalk, cutting away the kale from it. Place the whole leaves in a pan of boiling water with salt and let it boil, removing before it's overcooked and wilting. Drain very well and serve on a platter with lots of olive oil, lemon juice and plenty of sea salt. Add black pepper to taste.

Alternatively, you can chop the cavolo nero into pieces, toss in a pan of olive oil with chopped garlic and a little water and stir while it cooks. Serve with olive oil and lemon as above.

Lentils with pancetta

Serves 4

250g green lentils
Sea salt, to taste
Best-quality extra-virgin olive oil
50g pancetta, sliced
1 clove garlic, peeled and crushed
Large bunch of parsley, chopped

Boil the lentils in salted water until they are cooked but not soft helpful to last an indication of time about 20 minutes. Drain. In a deep frying pan, heat some olive oil and add the pancetta; cook for a minute or two. Add the lentils with the garlic and plenty of parsley. Mix all together over a medium-high heat until the lentils are covered in oil. Serve.

(For a vegetarian option simply leave out the pancetta.)

Epilogue

I am walking round an exhibition of Betsy's ceramics at a London gallery. Standing among the other exhibits is a triptych of long and lissom pots, covered in squiggles and flowers floating around a naked figure with big curly hair.

'*Amore*,' says Bernardo from behind me, 'that's your bottom!' I check the date on the work, and sure enough, it was made in 2008, the year I posed for Betsy. I remember that day, my despair over the dastardly Dino – an experience that inexorably brought me to this man, the one who is still by my side, the life partner who can spot a facsimile of my bottom at a hundred paces.

To allow Bernardo into my life I had to drop my prejudices, say yes a few times instead of no, and take a risk with my heart. Sometimes I think we have been so spoilt by the fairy tale that is continually sold to us – even as adults – that we fail to realise that true love is not an idealised romance that comes tied up with a Hollywood-style bow. Real love and real life, as my mother told me, is messy, imperfect, flawed – and so much better than I could have possibly imagined.

Much has changed in the decade since I encountered the *bella figura*, but I still drink my olive oil and I still walk as much, and as proudly, as possible (a study by Ohio University showed that the straighter you stand, the more confident you feel). I still honour each meal with attention (no screens) and a variety of courses, even if a course is just one radish or half a fennel. I have observed, with fascination, as the health fads and special diets I once followed have been replaced by clean-eating and the wellness movement. But I remain convinced that at the heart of being healthy, there must be pleasure involved: to eat well, we must enjoy what we eat. I continue to preach a sort of Italian moderation: home-cooked pasta and fresh vegetables are good for you if eaten the right way in the right quantities. I encourage spoonfuls of fresh extra-virgin olive oil and creamy cappuccinos with full-fat milk to start the day – although not at the same time, obviously. I am convinced that there is no true health possible if, while imbibing so much juiced – or rather nutritionally extracted – kale, one no longer enjoys actually eating; I am sure that no amount of spiralising can make up for the joylessness of deprivation, and that there are not enough gluten-free products in the world to counter the devastating effects of stress and giving no time at all to your inner self.

The food that is good for us has been good for us for thousands of years. Mostly, it is simple and unfussy. So, to that end, the *bella figura* way is not a diet. It's more about what we put into our bodies than what we don't. We detox our cupboards instead of ourselves, eliminating anything that doesn't bear any resemblance to its origins, anything with E-numbers and microwavable packaging and a sell-by date that exceeds our own expected lifetime. Those chemically reconstructed hydrogenated fats (trans fats) that are added to food to preserve their shelf life cannot be broken down by the body, entering the bloodstream where they clog arteries and damage blood-vessel linings, leading not just to weight gain, but also to cardiovascular diseases.

The thing about whole foods – food that acknowledges that it was once a potato or a fresh chicken – is that they won't do us any harm when eaten in balance and with variety. It's all very well popping supplements alongside ready-prepared meals, but nature intended us to eat the whole fish – the mackerel, the salmon, the sardine – not just an extract of its oil. Living the *bella figura* means we don't bastardise our foodstuffs and that we eat harmonious and well-balanced meals. Variety – and portion control – is key.

Of course, not many of us live in a shed in the middle of a market garden. We want to eat strawberries out of season and there is often only time for one weekly shop in our busy lives. But if we aim for the ideal, then we can deviate from it when necessary. And to deviate is normal. Above all, we must let go of the toxic notion of perfection and cherish the human we have been given to steer through this life – ourselves – and not bully, berate and belittle her if she fails sometimes.

The proliferation of farmers' markets makes fresh natural eating easier, but the humble greengrocer will do just as well. For many of us, though, it is impossible to fit this ideal into our daily lives, and it's OK to order a supermarket delivery online – just shop intelligently, and be sure to go for fresh and natural foods as much as possible.

Twice a year, for two months at a time, I walk back into the building from which I walked out clutching my redundancy cheque a decade ago. These days I take the stairs, but my ascent is no longer about avoiding the fashionistas in the lift; instead, it's about keeping my body moving. For those months, I am back at my editor's desk, a cog in the wheel of magazine creativity – and I could not love it more. I have learnt to appreciate what I am good at, and I don't sweat the rest. On my way to work, I get out a few stops early and walk through the park, waving to the giraffes who bat their pretty eyelashes at me. I take my own olive oil, coffee and lunch when I can. I make sure to decant my food on to a plate, drizzle with the fine olive oil I keep in the cupboard, and to set a place, even if it is in front of the computer.

But I leave my desk every day for a wander, for at least half an hour, a stroll, some gentle exercise and time away from the blinking screen. I get up as often as possible: sitting for prolonged periods of time is thought to lead to early death, not to mention making fat cells in the bottom more liable to expand. So I get up every fifteen minutes or so and move about for two minutes. My frequent walks over to colleagues' desks to ask something rather than emailing them helps prevent diabetes and heart disease.

The *bella figura* habit of smiling sincerely – at a colleague across the room, or a stranger walking down the street – provides precious instants of connection; momentary interactions that release endorphins. And that in turn helps banish cortisol and encourages stored belly fat to melt away – that and the extra-virgin olive oil which fights dangerous stomach fat, as evidenced by the wealth of research, such as the PERIMED study, which showed extra-virgin olive oil reduces risk of cardiovascular disease, diabetes and insulin sensitivity. Scientists at Reina Sofia University Hospital in Cordoba, Spain found that in just four weeks of replacing other fats with extra-virgin olive oil, both visceral and deep belly fat was reduced; both the *British Journal of Medicine* and the American Diabetes Association have published studies confirming this. It comes as no surprise to me that the Bloomberg Global Health Index recently put Italy at the top of its list of the world's healthiest countries.

I have learnt to embrace the world around me. When I am in Florence, most Sunday mornings you can fnd me sitting in the choir pew of the English church, fanning away the plumes of incense smoke that scratch my throat. I sing under the frescoes next to plaques in honour of the Keppels and their daughter Violet Trefusis, a reminder that countless Brits have been seduced by Florence's beauty and the Italian lifestyle. As well as the joy of singing and ritual, I cherish my time with the other choristers, and the space early on Sunday mornings between rehearsal and the service when we all go for a coffee together.

They form one of the many communities I am a part of, and, like a Venn diagram, these different groups all have one thing in common: they provide connection and relationship, one of the most important elements of the *bella figura* lifestyle.

Considering the difference between the Italian way of life – with its squares thronging with all the generations and the nightly *passeggiata* – and our own northern European/American tendency to live as solo a life as possible, it is perhaps no surprise that Italy's suicide rate is far lower than our own (according to research published by the WHO in 2015, 5.4 out of 100,000 people committed suicide per year in Italy, whereas the rate in the United States was 12.6 out of 100,000) and that in the UK in 2016, 64.7 million antidepressant prescriptions were given out – double that of a decade ago. Unsurprisingly, loneliness adversely affects the immune and cardiovascular systems and has been proven to be worse for one's health than smoking. To be healthy we need to see our friends and family, visit our grannies, call up our aunts and cousins. And a phone call is better than a text message – a radical claim these days when communication by emoji is ubiquitous, but hearing a loved one's voice can be just as comforting if it is not possible to see them in person. So let's go back to doing things together, even if it's just a stroll in the park or a visit to the greengrocer. It may just save our lives.

Today, whether we're in Tuscany or London, Bernardo and I shop at the market (and even the supermarket) together, we cook simple multiple-course meals and, when we come to London for an extended period, we bring over five-litre tins of green extra-virgin olive oil, much as the Italian immigrants used to when they returned from visiting Italy. My family has expanded once more to include children, dogs, even Bernardo's ex-wives. Most of all, we take care of each other. At my father's funeral, Bernardo bore his coffin on his shoulders; months later I held carefully the still-warm ashes of his mother in my hands as we drove her for the final time back to her castle from the crematorium. How we have navigated these years owes much to the *bella figura*: the trials and tribulations of being a stepmother, settling into life in the Tuscan countryside and the struggle to span both our countries, families, dreams and goals have been infinitely helped by what I learnt in Florence that first year. Most of all, how to be kind to myself, how to treat my own human with the same love and care reserved for a beloved friend, even when rebellious teens and jealous exes did not. But then, that is a whole other story.

HOW TO BRING THE *BELLA FIGURA* HOME

- Drink a spoonful of excellent-quality extra-virgin olive oil four times a day.
- Get your coffee to stay! Make sure it is of excellent quality and forget the to-go cup.
- Eat the best-quality whole fruits, vegetables, meats and cheeses that you can find.
- Find bread that is made from unadulterated wheat. Many people with gluten allergies find they have no such problems with bread in Italy.

- The food that you eat should give you pleasure while eating it.
- Wherever you are, pause for meals, lay a proper place and turn off all screens.
- Eliminate all ready-meals and anything with E-numbers. Read labels, get informed.
- Seek out your community; don't be fooled by the remote connection offered by social media.
- Seize any opportunity to get moving – be it taking the stairs, doing the coffee run at work, or hoovering with gusto.
- Find a form of exercise that you love. Bring it into your daily routine. Go to the gym only if it makes your heart actually sing.
- Better still join a dance class: learning a new skill burns new pathways in your brain, and releases those feel-good hormones. It will give you a community, a new passion, have music pumping through your body (instead of cortisol) and dancing in hold will give you some of those ten embraces a day that scientists say release oxytocin and make you feel loving and compassionate.
- Stay hydrated but do not carry one of those toxic little plastic bottles of water around and do not drink on the go. Go into a café and spend a few minutes drinking water from a glass. Keep a jug of water on your desk.
- Drink alcohol in moderation – a small glass of wine with dinner is your guide. A report suggests it is women with expensive homes and six-figure

salaries who drink more than any other social group: up to two-thirds will drink more than the healthy limit. The *bella figura* demands we break this unhealthy relationship with alcohol. Remember that drinking to excess will pile on weight and stress out your skin as well as all the internal damage it is doing.

- Walk with style. Good posture is all-important. Walk tall as if offering your heart up to the sky.

- Look up more, and smile much more. Looking down at our smartphones is leading to early ageing – slackening our jawlines prematurely, sagging our faces, giving us jowls way before they are due.

- Seek out nature, be it a city park, a tree on your street or some wild place.

- Slow down! Climbing stairs deliberately instead of running up them two at a time has been proven to lose you an extra pound a month.

- Love yourself. Remember the Italian woman – the *Bella Figura* – occupies her space, emotionally and physically, with God-given entitlement. Nurture and protect your human – she's the only one you have and has been entrusted to your care.

- Be graceful. Mind your manners, be courteous and respect your elders.

- Seek connection. Return calls, reply to texts and emails, be reliable.

- Be happy, you always have the choice.

ACKNOWLEDGEMENTS

If all ideas begin with a spark, then this one ignited on a dark winter night in London in a magazine office where I was working late. And the spark came not to me but to a colleague whose face literally lit up as she envisaged not just the book and the story, but the title itself. So my first thanks must go to the brilliant Farrah Storr who, in that moment of inspiration, introduced me to *Bella Figura*, my new book.

The idea was developed through conversations and research with Clare Naylor who gave up chunks of her summer holiday to help shape the proposal. This book would not exist without her and *Bella* will always belong just as much to Clare as to me.

The nascent idea was nurtured by my agent Judith Murray in London who tirelessly read various drafts, and by Grainne Fox, my agent in NYC, whose kick-ass enthusiasm has lifted *Bella* out of many a slump; my thanks and appreciation go to them both.

Alexandra Pringle, my editor at Bloomsbury, embodies all the grace and beauty of the true *Bella Figura*, and her wise words have carried me along the years and through the low points. I can hardly find the words to express my love and gratitude. In the US, my editor Lexy Bloom has been an unfailing supporter and has helped guide the story with her astute comments and vision. Big thanks also to Faiza Khan of Bloomsbury whose inspiringly bold edits drove the book through the final stages.

All writers should be so lucky to have such incredible women on-side.

Thanks, as always, go to my family: my late father, my mother and my sister; my base and foundation in everything I do. Also to Kicca Tommasi who was my first reader, and Grayson Splane who introduced me to the cookbooks of Artusi. Of course I am beyond indebted to Christobel Kent who sent me to Florence and thus changed my life, and to my Florentine family who made arriving in their city just like coming home.

Thanks to my *amore* Bernardo Conti, whose love enriches my life, and who has patiently borne all the different versions of 'writing retreat' he has had to live with. *Grazie amore* for the chaos and the kids and the dogs and the puppies and also for bringing me such delicious meals on a tray when I couldn't tear myself away.

The biggest thanks must go to Florence herself, this luminous love of my life who continues to uplift me with her golden light and extraordinary beauty, and the many flavours of her *gelato*.

A NOTE ON THE AUTHOR

Kamin Mohammadi was born in Iran in 1969 and exiled to the UK in 1979. She is an experienced journalist, writer and broadcaster who has written for *The Times,* the *Financial Times*, *Harper's Bazaar*, *Marie Claire* and the *Guardian*, and has appeared as a commentator on various BBC, Channel Four and American radio stations. Her first book, *The Cypress Tree*, was published in 2011. Kamin Mohammadi currently lives in Italy.

www.kamin.co.uk

A NOTE ON THE TYPE

The text of this book is set in Perpetua. This typeface is an adaptation of a style of letter that had been popularised for monumental work in stone by Eric Gill. Large-scale drawings by Gill were given to Charles Malin, a Parisian punch-cutter, and his hand-cut punches were the basis for the font issued by Monotype. First used in a private translation called 'The Passion of Perpetua and Felicity', the italic was originally called Felicity.